T5-CQQ-487

Contemporary Diagnosis, Prevention, and Management of
Influenza®

Arnold S. Monto, MD
Professor of Epidemiology
University of Michigan School of Public Health
Ann Arbor, Michigan

Second Edition

Published by Handbooks in Health Care Co.,
Newtown, Pennsylvania, USA

This book has been prepared and is presented as a service to the medical community. The information provided reflects the knowledge, experience, and personal opinions of the author, Arnold S. Monto, MD, Professor, Department of Epidemiology, University of Michigan School of Public Health, Ann Arbor, Michigan.

This book is not intended to replace or to be used as a substitute for the complete prescribing information prepared by each manufacturer for each drug. Because of possible variations in drug indications, in dosage information, in newly described toxicities, in drug/drug interactions, and in other items of importance, reference to such complete prescribing information is definitely recommended before any of the drugs discussed are used or prescribed.

International Standard Book Number: 978-1-931981-92-7

Library of Congress Catalog Card Number: 2005937752

Table of Contents

Chapter **1**

Introduction

Influenza has a long history of documented outbreaks. Yet it is a disease that is sometimes poorly understood not only in the media, but also in the biomedical profession. Flu outbreaks are often reported in the press during the summer and, on further examination, are identified as gastroenteric illness. Now there is confusion between avian influenza in humans and regular seasonal influenza.

Influenza can be tracked over the centuries because its characteristics and its occurrence in the population are easy to recognize. The seasonal outbreaks of disease can be large, with the typical syndrome including a respiratory illness with fever, cough, and systemic symptoms. However, the major impact of this disease, in terms of mortality, disruption, and cost, has only gradually been appreciated. It was recognized for a time following the 1918 Spanish flu pandemic, but memories have been short. Now, awareness is changing globally, and even in the developing world, influenza is being given its due as a cause of preventable mortality. The development and introduction of new interventions to prevent and treat influenza, as well as a new pandemic threat, have also helped increase recognition.

This handbook covers many aspects of the influenza story. Because influenza produces not only annual epidemics, but also sometimes devastating pandemics, its history must be taken into account. It has been more than 30 years since the last true pandemic, so another one is long overdue. The 1997 bird flu in Hong Kong was a wake-up call to remind the world of what could happen again. Since late 2003, avian influenza has returned and has continued to spread, but has not yet become able to transmit efficiently from person to person. History can and will repeat itself, so the past must not be ignored.

The influenza viruses are unique in their ability to change through two different behaviors known as 'shift' and 'drift.' However, in order to understand these phenomena, the virus must be examined; the way the vaccines and antivirals act depends on the virus and its structure. Immunity to influenza infection is critical to understanding why, even if the virus does not change, we still have to give the inactivated vaccine annually in order to get adequate protection. The protection of the vaccine is short-lived, partly because of changes in antigen.

Influenza in its uncomplicated form is now well recognized. However, some of the complications are rarely seen and need to be remembered; paradoxically, other complications have not been previously related to influenza because of their frequent occurrence. For example, otitis media, which is common in children, has been significantly reduced by influenza vaccine and antivirals, documenting that it is a complication of influenza in children.

Influenza outbreaks vary according to the type or subtype of virus causing them, which can differ with each season. Some epidemics produce major outbreaks in schools but little illness in adults; others result in deaths in the elderly. Epidemiologic surveillance documents these patterns.

New methods of laboratory diagnosis have been developed in recent years. Many offer significant advantages over past tests in terms of their simplicity and rapidity. Questions have been raised regarding sacrifices made for this simplicity, and how and when to use these tests. These methods do have a role in the future, but it may be a smaller one than some people think.

Type A influenza infects various mammals and birds, as well as humans. This is important because there is much evidence that the last two pandemics have come from the reassortment of human and avian viruses. The 1918 pandemic virus was also avian in origin, and became able to infect humans by mutation. Surveillance in these species and in humans who have contact with them may help with earlier recognition of the next pandemic virus. Therefore, awareness of the ecology of influenza viruses is beneficial.

Vaccines for influenza have been available since World War II, when they were used to keep the military ready for combat. The inactivated vaccine is effective in preventing influenza in healthy adults and in preventing complications and death in older individuals. Recommendations for use often change, and will change even more when the live intranasal vaccine becomes available and is administered to new population groups.

The antivirals amantadine (Symmetrel®) and rimantadine (Flumadine®) have been available for many years and have been useful in prophylaxis and in the treatment of influenza. A marked increase in resistance has rendered their use problematic. The new neuraminidase inhibitors offer significant advantages, including their ability to prevent complications. This advantage applies particularly to special populations, such as the immunocompromised and nursing home residents. Future pandemics will produce special challenges in which vaccines and antivirals will need to be used together. Planning is critical so that response can be rapid. This planning has accelerated with reports of occasional spread of 'bird flu' to humans.

This handbook covers all of these topics and attempts to provide answers to critical questions. It also attempts to guide decision making. However, it can only be a guide to a complex subject. The reader is urged to look further to the original publications cited and the suggested readings. In this way, this handbook will provide a road map to learning more about influenza and its control.

Chapter 2

History: Lessons From the Past

There are few infectious diseases that can be traced back in history in the same way as influenza. One infectious disease, rabies, has been identified for millennia; in fact, the dog star, Sirius, was given its name because it reaches its peak in the summer, when rabid dogs were typically the most abundant. Another example is poliomyelitis, which can be traced back to ancient Egypt, where mummies have been discovered with shortened limbs that are almost certainly a result of paralysis. Similarly, some have attempted to trace influenza back to ancient Greece. The 'Plague of Athens,' which has been speculated to have been influenza with bacterial complications, had a major historic role in the decline of that city.[1]

However, many agree that the first clear description of influenza as we now recognize it was the arrival of the so-called 'newe acquayantance' in the Scottish court, as reported in 1562 by the Ambassador of Queen Elizabeth I of England.[2] The term is an interesting one because it reflects the idea that an influenza pandemic is somehow novel. Each time that a pandemic has occurred in the past century, it has been treated as a unique event, with the basic facts about influenza being rediscovered. The disease occurrence reported in Scotland in 1562, with fever, coughing, and systemic symptoms, is comparable with what we now recognize as typical influenza. The fact that the syndrome is typical and that the outbreaks have been large has allowed for the recognition of outbreaks as influenza, even without virologic confirmation.

Early Pandemics

Influenza historians have identified possible pandemics between the 16th century and the later 19th century. However, the extent of these pandemics is subject to some debate because only partial information is available. That is not the case with the pandemic that involved the United States in 1889-1890, following a long period of relative quiescence of influenza activity. This was a true pandemic, with severe outbreaks reported in the United Kingdom as well. Good data are available from the state of Massachusetts, and they establish the age-specific patterns of mortality, typical for every major outbreak to the present with one major exception. This pattern is summarized in the saying, "Many sicken but few die." In other words, despite the extensive morbidity in healthy children and adults, deaths are concentrated at the extremes of age, especially in children younger than 2 years, with even more in children younger than 1 year, and in older individuals.

A new virus may have begun to circulate around 1900, but there are no records of typical large-scale outbreaks, at least not in the United States and Western Europe.[3] However, in the autumn of 1918, many did sicken, as is typical in a pandemic of a new influenza virus, but many also died.[4] It was not only those at the extremes of age, but also healthy, young adults who died rapidly of hemorrhagic pneumonia and bacterial complications. These outbreaks took place at the end of World War I, but it was not only the military that was involved. Stories abound about individuals or couples living in remote farm houses, who, having not been heard from, were found to be dead or profoundly ill and unable to care for themselves. The episode was, at the time, referred to as Spanish influenza, probably because, unlike other countries, Spain, as a nonparticipant in the war, did not have censorship in place to conceal the magnitude of the disaster. Features of this pandemic, which could be related to what is now recognized as the swine influenza virus, are used as the worst-case scenario in current pandemic plans. Such plans try to anticipate phenomena experienced in 1918, such as the lack of necessary hospital beds, medical personnel, and even burial facilities. When the impact of this health catastrophe was originally quantified, it was estimated that 500,000 individuals had died in the United States and 20 million individuals had died worldwide. As a result of more recent studies, the worldwide number has been doubled, or even tripled, because most of what is now considered the developing world was omitted in the original count. The impact of this pandemic was even greater in these developing countries because of the lack of any supportive medical care. Pandemics of influenza do not skip any part of the world.

The 1918 flu pandemic was accompanied by and followed by major, but unsuccessful, efforts to identify the etiologic agent involved. This has, in fact, continued up to the present, with the entire genome of the virus recently sequenced and reconstructed from tissue frozen in exhumed bodies or preserved as pathologic specimens.[5] However, these studies have still not fully answered the basic question: why was this virus so lethal? Recent data indicate that multiple genes of the virus itself were responsible. At the time, there were some who thought that the bacterium *Haemophilus influenzae*, previously misidentified as the cause of influenza, was at least partially involved.

The virus that causes human influenza was not identified until the 1930s, and, surprisingly, it was first identified in animals, an indirect result of work being done in the United Kingdom on canine distemper.[6] At that time, puppies in England were experiencing a continuing outbreak of distemper, and it was discovered that ferrets, which were used to hunt field pests, were susceptible to the distemper virus. A syndrome similar to human influenza, including fever, was produced when the ferrets were inoculated with secretions from someone with influenza. One problem was that it had proven hard to distinguish between influenza and distemper in the ferrets. That problem was solved when an infected ferret sneezed onto Sir Charles Stuart-Harris. Distemper does not affect humans, and Sir Charles, by developing influenza, demonstrated that the virus being propagated in the ferrets was the one causing human influenza.[7] Similar studies were conducted in the United States by Thomas Francis, Jr., who identified a similar virus, confirming that this was the cause of influenza all over the world.[8]

The ferret was a cumbersome tool for primary isolation of any virus. Fortunately, research using fertilized hens' eggs had been ongoing, and it was soon discovered that the influenza virus replicated in this host. This discovery had implications not only for the ability to more accurately identify the virus, but also for vaccine production. Another important development, which was somewhat related, was the discovery that the virus agglutinated red blood cells of various species.[9] This agglutination could be specifically prevented by antibody, allowing serologic studies to be performed.

In 1940, a virus was reported that was distinct from the one previously identified. This new virus was named type B, and those seen before were termed type A.[10] The type B virus causes a typical influenza syndrome, unlike the virus that was identified as type C. The type C virus did not cause an influenza-like illness and, in addition, required very careful inoculation of eggs to isolate. Nearly all work done with influenza thereafter is concerned with type A and B viruses. Far fewer studies have been conducted on the type C virus, which most commonly causes a syndrome similar to the common cold.

When it became possible to compare strains using the hemagglutination inhibition test, it became clear that influenza viruses were not antigenically stable, but changed gradually from year to year. Further diversity was recognized when isolates from various animals, such as pigs, were documented. In fact, the virus that causes swine influenza was the first of such viruses isolated in the United States. The other group of viruses that cause clinical influenza in mammals was identified much later, along with the profusion of influenza viruses in various types of domestic and wild birds. Recent reports of influenza in seals and other animals confirm the diversity of influenza.

Development of Influenza Vaccines

Soon after the discovery of type B influenza, the first influenza vaccine was developed, following a few short-lived efforts in the United Kingdom. The impetus was World War II and the realization that an influenza outbreak could affect military readiness by simultaneously incapacitating significant numbers of troops. An effective approach to producing the vaccine was growing the virus in embryonated eggs and then using formalin to inactivate the virus. The same technique continues to be used for vaccine production, with improved concentration of virus and greater removal of impurities, such as egg proteins. Under the Armed Forces Commission on Influenza, controlled clinical trials were conducted on an annual basis, with the repeated finding that vaccine is 70% to 90% efficacious in preventing laboratory-confirmed influenza.[11] From time to time, variations, such as the addition of adjuvants, were attempted. Another observation made during this period was that, if the circulating influenza viruses changed between seasons, the vaccine that was formulated with the virus from the previous season would be only partially effective.

Influenza Viruses: A Moving Target

Until 1947, the influenza vaccine continued to be effective on an annual basis, but in the winter of 1946-1947, it had no efficacy in preventing against illness caused by a type A virus. At the time, it was thought that a major antigenic change in the virus had occurred; however, there was not a total change in either of the two surface antigens, the hemagglutinin or the neuraminidase. One indication that a total change, what we now call a shift, had not taken place was the lack of a resulting pandemic. However, the terminology used at the time was changed; viruses isolated before 1947 were called A0 and those isolated after 1947 were called A prime or A1.

In 1957, the first pandemic of influenza in the era of modern virology occurred. The outbreak started in central China early in the year, but because of political conditions, it was not recognized until outbreaks began in Hong Kong in April, spreading rapidly throughout East Asia.[12] The virus was quickly identified to be different from the A1 viruses that had been the prevalent type A virus up to that time, and it was named A2 or Asian Influenza. In the United States, sporadic cases began in early June. An international meeting was held in Grinell, IA, in late June, and 200 cases occurred there, with participants subsequently returning to all parts of the country. In August, outbreaks were documented in Louisiana, where schools were already open, and by September, outbreaks were occurring throughout the country. By that time, it was clear that the disease occurrence was not like 1918; there were deaths, but mainly in older individuals and the very young. However, there was still extensive, major morbidity in all age groups. The deaths were carefully studied, and autopsies were performed on a significant number of cases. An unusual finding was that individuals with underlying rheumatic heart disease, particularly with mitral stenosis, fared poorly and experienced a primary viral pneumonia with a tremendous exudation of fluid into the lungs.[13] However, in the general population, bacterial complications were more commonly experienced, and with the emergence of antibiotic-resistant staphylococci, such cases were frequently reported. In this pandemic, an elevated frequency of pneumonia in pregnant women was also reported. This observation, along with more recent data, has resulted in a change in recommendations for annual administration of vaccine to include pregnant women.[14] Overall, it was conservatively estimated that at least 40,000 people died in the first wave of this pandemic, which killed 80,000 Americans in the second wave.

Both surface antigens, the hemagglutinin and the neuraminidase, changed in 1957 as a result of reassortment with avian viruses. In the next few years, these viruses, along with type B viruses, caused regular, annual influenza outbreaks. The type A viruses from before 1957 disappeared completely. Eleven years later, a major outbreak of influenza was again recognized, first in Hong Kong, after earlier spread in China. The Hong Kong outbreak took place in July and early August over the course of approximately 6 weeks (Figure 1). Isolated cases occurred in the continental United States from late August to mid-October. Thereafter, the virus spread mainly from west to east, peaking during December. At that time, very small amounts of vaccine were available, but they were mainly for experimental use. The impact was major, but less severe than the impact of the 1957 episode. This may be because only the hemagglutinin and not the neuraminidase of the virus had changed. It is clear that this virus came from an avian source. This new virus replaced the old A2 virus and was initially termed the Hong Kong virus.

The hemagglutinin of the 1968 virus is now recognized as an 'H3.' In fact, the modern classification of hemagglutinin and neuraminidase was hastened by this event. The first classification system attempted to identify hemagglutinin and neuraminidase by the animal source of the viruses. For example, the virus derived from pigs, which was related to the one that caused the 1918 pandemic, was called Hsw1, with 'sw' standing for swine. However, the close resemblance in molecular structure between the human and the swine H1 viruses persuaded the classifiers that it was not possible to separate the type A virus hemagglutinin

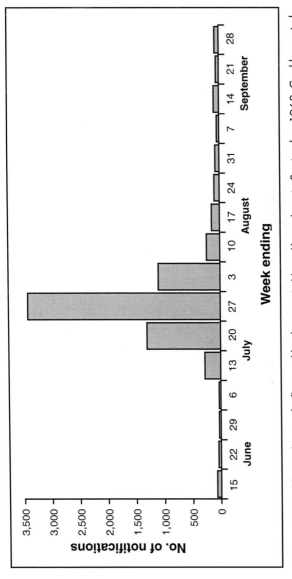

Figure 1: Weekly incidence of influenza-like diseases in Hong Kong, June to September 1968. Cockburn et al, *Bull World Health Organ* 1969;41:345-348.

and neuraminidase by species of origin. Eventually, the hemagglutinins of all species were numbered from 1 to 16, and the neuraminidases were numbered from 1 to 9. The human viruses of 1918 through 1956 resembled each other molecularly and were designated H1N1. This molecular relationship explained why the change in viruses in 1947 did not produce a true pandemic. The Asian virus of 1957 was designated H2N2, and the 1968 Hong Kong virus was designated H3N2.

The Swine Influenza Nonpandemic, 1976

The swine version of the type A(H1N1) virus is known to circulate in pigs in the United States and in many other countries. This virus, or one related to it, was thought at the time to have caused the 1918 pandemic. One theory of influenza pandemics is that the A subtypes cycle, with one following the other. As shown in Table 1, it was thought possible that an A(H1N1) virus might produce the next pandemic. Therefore, when an outbreak of influenza occurred among military recruits in Fort Dix, NJ, in early 1976, and the cause was found to be a swine-like influenza virus, it provoked a sense of alarm.[15] A new or returned influenza virus had never before been transmitted in outbreak form, from person to person, without a pandemic following, and this virus resembled that of the catastrophic pandemic of 1918. Therefore, only in the United States, a major national effort was organized to prepare for a possible pandemic. This mainly involved the development of a monovalent vaccine for the type A New Jersey virus, H1N1, which caused the Fort Dix outbreak, but it also included surveillance. However, vaccine production became complicated by nonscientific issues when the manufacturers demanded liability protection that had to be approved by Congress.

Thereafter, major studies were launched to determine how many doses of vaccine would be required, as well as to determine the minimum amount of antigen that would

Table 1:	History of Human Type A Influenza Hemagglutinins	
Year	Hemagglutinin	Name of Outbreak
1889	H2	—
1900	H3	Pandemic not confirmed*
1918	H1	Spanish or swine influenza
1957	H2	Asian influenza
1968	H3	Hong Kong influenza
1977	H1	Russian influenza, age limited

be required per dose; this was important to extend the vaccine's availability. Although no further transmittal of the virus was documented, the vaccine program began, with the plan of making the vaccine available to all who wanted it. A special vaccine that also contained the type A(H3N2) virus was formulated for individuals in the traditional high-risk group because this virus was also circulating. The program was abruptly terminated when reports began to accumulate about a possible relation of swine influenza vaccination to Guillain-Barré syndrome. This episode, while yielding a great deal of information on how vaccine could be used, probably had a more negative long-term impact on efforts to control influenza because it involved an apparent loss of credibility.

More Recent Developments

Thereafter, the type A(H3N2) and type B viruses circulated. In 1977, 'Russian influenza,' as it was termed at the time, appeared. However, it did not start in the former Soviet Union; it had already been spreading in China for many months. Unlike previous pandemic viruses, which showed molecular similarity to avian viruses, this virus, identified as an A(H1N1) subtype, closely resembled a well-characterized human virus that had been isolated in the United States in 1950. Another peculiarity was that this virus did not significantly infect anyone older than 20 to 25 years (ie, anyone who had experienced the previously circulating A(H1N1) viruses). Also, before 1977, whenever a new type A virus appeared, it always replaced the previous type A virus. For example, in 1968, after new type A(H3N2) viruses emerged, the A(H2N2) virus was no longer isolated. However, this was not the case in 1977. Since that time, both the returned A(H1N1) virus and the A(H3N2) virus have circulated, so both viruses must be included in the vaccine. Because of the similarity of the A(H1N1) virus, which caused the 1977-1978 outbreak, to a 1950 isolate, it has been hypothesized that its reemergence might be related to the extensive human experimentation with a potential vaccine, but there are no concrete data to support this theory.

Since 1977, there have been no new pandemics. However, in 1997, there was a major scare when an avian virus, A(H5N1), which probably came from a goose, produced lethal infections in the live-bird market in Hong Kong.[16] In theory, that avian virus could not spread from birds to humans because of the difference in receptors; however, it did spread, with 18 documented cases in humans. The disease was severe in adults of all ages, with six deaths. This suggests dissemination of the virus and multisystem involvement, which is extremely rare in human influenza. The disease appeared to be worse than the influenza of 1918 in terms of lethality; however, this virus, while able to spread from chicken to human, did not effectively spread from human to human. When the A(H3N2) virus appeared in Hong Kong and started to spread in humans, there was concern that, if the episode was not stopped, the A(H5N1) avian virus might recombine with the human virus and be transformed into one that could spread more effectively. Therefore, a decision was made to 'depopulate' the bird markets. The virus has returned throughout much of East and Southeast Asia, and now Europe and Africa; occasional human cases have continued. This situation is addressed in some detail in Chapter 15.

References

1. Langmuir AD, Worthen TD, Solomon J, et al: The Thucydides syndrome. A new hypothesis for the cause of the plague of Athens. *New Engl J Med* 1985;313:1027-1030.

2. Francis T Jr: Influenza: The newe acquayatance. *Ann Intern Med* 1953;39:203-221.

3. Masurel N, Marine WM: Recycling of Asian and Hong Kong influenza A virus hemagglutinins in man. *Am J Epidemiol* 1973;97: 44-49.

4. MacNeal WJ: The influenza epidemic of 1918 in the American Expeditionary Forces in France and England. *Arch Intern Med* 1918; 23:657-688.

5. Taubenberger JK, Reid AH, Lourens RM, et al: Characterization of the 1918 influenza virus polymerase genes. *Nature* 2005;437: 889-893.

6. Smith W, Andrewes CH, Laidlaw PP: A virus obtained from influenza patients. *Lancet* 1933;2:66-68.

7. Smith W, Stuart-Harris CH: Influenza infection of man from the ferret. *Lancet* 1936;2:121-123.

8. Francis T Jr: Transmission of influenza by a filterable virus. *Science* 1934;80:457-459.

9. Hirst GK: The agglutination of red cells by allantoic fluid of chick embryos infected with influenza virus. *Science* 1941;94: 22-23.

10. Francis T Jr: A new type of virus from epidemic influenza. *Science* 1940;92:405-406.

11. Francis T Jr, Salk JE, Brace WM: The protective effect of vaccination against influenza B. *JAMA* 1946;131:275-278.

12. Dunn FL: Pandemic influenza in 1957. *Am J Med Assoc* 1958; 166:1140-1148.

13. Burch GE, Walsh JJ, Mogabgab W: A study of the response of the cardiovascular system to Asian influenza. *Am Rev Respir Dis* 1961;83:68-78.

14. Freeman DW, Barno A: Deaths from Asian influenza associated with pregnancy. *Am J Obstet Gynecol* 1959;78:1172-1175.

15. Top FH Jr, Russell PK: Swine influenza A at Fort Dix, New Jersey (January-February 1976). IV. Summary and speculation. *J Infect Dis* 1977;136:S376-S380.

16. Subbarao K, Klimov A, Katz J, et al: Characterization of an avian influenza A(H5N1) virus isolated from a child with a fatal respiratory illness. *Science* 1998;279:393-396.

Chapter 3

Virology

Types of Influenza Viruses

The viruses that cause influenza have been alphabetically named in the order of their identification: influenza types A, B, and C. These viruses are three genera within the family of orthomyxoviruses. In addition to human hosts, influenza A viruses infect avian species, swine, and horses; influenza B and C viruses have only been isolated from humans. Influenza type A viruses exist as multiple antigenically distinct subtypes based on variations in the two viral envelope glycoproteins, hemagglutinin (HA) and neuraminidase (NA). Of these multiple subtypes, only H1N1, H2N2, and H3N2 have been isolated from epidemic human infections. Influenza types B and C lack subtypes, perhaps as a result of their single host species. Minor antigenic variations in the surface glycoproteins of all three influenza types occur sequentially with time and result in strain variation among circulating types and subtypes. New strains, detected as a result of annual epidemiologic surveillance, are designated by type, place of original isolation, isolate number, year of isolation, and subtype (in type A viruses [eg, A/California/07/2004(H3N2)]). Type C does not cause epidemic disease and, therefore, is rarely encountered; however, it does cause a syndrome similar to a common cold. Variations in circulating type, subtype, and strain type are responsible for the epidemiologic patterns of recurring infection and disease associated with influenza. Neutralizing antibodies to specific HA and NA glycoproteins develop after infection or vaccination and may provide protection from future illness. Designations of predominant or new circulating strains are relevant to vaccine formulation because variation may reduce vaccine effectiveness. However, these are understandable only with reference to antigenic relationships determined in neutralization tests or, more usually, in hemagglutination inhibition tests. Sequencing of amino acids, particularly the HA and, to a lesser extent, the NA has also been valuable in comparing different viruses of the same type or subtype.

Viral Structure and Composition: Surface and Internal Antigens

Influenza viruses are heterogeneous in size and shape (pleomorphic), but are roughly spherical, filamentous particles with a diameter of 80 to 120 nm. The nucleic acid is negative-sense single-stranded RNA occurring as eight segments in influenza types A and B and as seven segments in influenza C. Each RNA segment is encapsidated by the viral nucleoprotein (NP) and, along with polymerase, forms the ribonucleoprotein (RNP) particles or nucleocapsid. The nucleocapsids are located within a layer of M1 proteins that line the lipid envelope derived from the infected host cell. In influenza A and B viruses, multiple spikes of the two surface glycoproteins, HA and NA, plus, in influenza A, the membrane-channel protein M2, project from this lipid membrane (see Figure 1).

The eight gene segments of influenza A and B viruses code for 10 proteins. Four segments code for the components of the RNA polymerase—PB1, PB2, PA, and the NP; all are involved in transcription and replication of the nucleic acid. The NP is antigenically stable and determines influenza type (A, B, or C). In influenza A and B, two gene segments code for the HA (a trimer of identical subunits) and NA (a tetramer). HA is responsible for receptor binding and membrane fusion, and NA is responsible for receptor-destroying activities. Influenza C has a single gene segment that codes for a single surface glycoprotein,

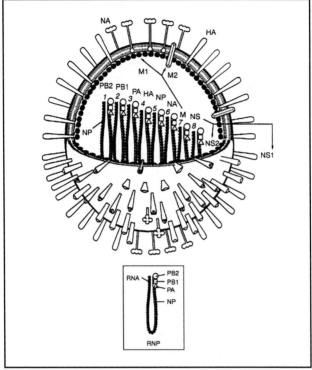

Figure 1: Schematic diagram of an influenza A virion. The virion contains hemagglutinin and neuraminidase spikes in addition to a third membrane protein, M2. Within the viral envelope are ribonucleoprotein (RNP), consisting of RNA segments associated with nucleoprotein and the PA, PB1, and PB2 polymerase proteins. Three polymerase proteins are associated with RNP at its end (insert). The precise location of M1 in virions is unknown, although it is associated with the virion envelope, RNP, and NS2. Cox NJ, Kawaoka Y: Orthomyxoviruses: influenza. In: Collier L, Balows A, Sussman M, eds: *Topley and Wilson's Microbiology and Microbial Infections. Volume 1: Virology.* 9th ed. London: Arnold, 1998, p. 388. Reproduced by permission of Arnold.

the hemagglutinin-esterase-fusion protein, which performs activities similar to the HA and NA of influenza A and B. In influenza B, the gene coding for NA also codes for NB, another component of the virus envelope, which may have a function in virus uncoating, similar to the M2 protein of influenza A. The M1 matrix protein is the major internal structural component of the virus particle; it exhibits antigenic stability similar to that of the NP. The M2 matrix protein is a membrane protein that forms an ion channel, which participates with the HA in the uncoating of an infecting virus. The antiviral activity of amantadine (Symmetrel®) and rimantadine (Flumadine®) suggests that the M2 protein is the likely site of replication inhibition in influenza A. This means that its activity is required for type A viruses, but not for type B. Two nonstructural proteins, NS1 and NS2, are also encoded in the virus. NS1 has various regulatory roles in virus replication, and NS2 has poorly understood roles, also in replication.

Virus Replication

Cellular infection is initiated by attachment of viral HA to cell-surface receptors containing N-acetyl-neuraminic acid (sialic acid) with $\alpha2,6$ linkage to galactose-containing oligosaccharides (see Figure 2). Humans, ferrets, and pigs possess this receptor; birds do not. A neutralizing antibody to specific HA will prevent this step. Following attachment, the virus enters the cell by receptor-mediated endocytosis (cellular uptake in endosomes). Virus uncoating and the entry of virion RNP into cellular cytoplasm occur as a result of a structural change in HA, resulting in membrane fusion and M2 ion channel (pH modulating activity) dependent dissociation of the M1 matrix protein from RNP. Transcription and replication of the viral genome occur in the nucleus of the virus-infected cell. Because influenza viruses are negative-strand RNA viruses, the virion contains RNA-dependent enzymes—the PB1, PB2, and PA proteins—required for transcription and

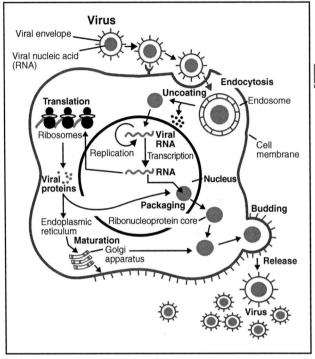

Figure 2: Process of viral replication. *Workshop on Antiviral Agents for Pandemic Influenza.* March 6-7, 2001; Atlanta, GA. Department of Health and Human Services.

replication of its genome. During primary transcription, virion RNA is transcribed into message-sense RNA. This process is followed by the synthesis of viral proteins and the replication of viral RNA. Nucleocapsids are assembled in the nucleus and migrate to the cell membrane. The M1 matrix protein becomes associated with the cell plasma membrane and virus membrane proteins, including the HA and NA glycoproteins, and the M2 proteins are inserted. Virion assembly takes place at the plasma membrane, and progeny viruses are released by budding at sites of altered cell membrane. The surface glycoproteins of newly synthesized virions contain cellular sialic acid (influenza virus receptor site). A major function of viral NA is enzymatic removal of these sialic acid residues to increase the number of infectious virus particles and replication cycles by preventing viral aggregates. Neutralizing antibodies to the NA glycoproteins will reduce the number of infectious virions. This activity is also the target of zanamivir (Relenza®) and oseltamivir (Tamiflu®). Vaccines contain HA and NA but are standardized only in terms of their HA content; antibodies to both, especially the more abundant HA, prevent viral replication.

The consequences of influenza infection for host cells are damage and, ultimately, destruction as host cell protein synthesis is inhibited and progeny viruses are synthesized. As progeny viruses are released, they infect adjacent cells. As a result, many cells in the respiratory tract become infected, release progeny viruses, and die. Host cell damage is demonstrated in tissue culture as 'cytopathic effect,' where infected cells are rounded and refractile, or is demonstrated by the formation of plaques that appear as visible areas of clearing, the result of cell lysis. The human host response to this process is characterized by fever, malaise, myalgia, cough, nasal obstruction, and sneezing. Many of these events are a result of the production of proinflammatory cytokines. These may have a particularly important role in avian influenza infections of humans.

Molecular Basis of Antigenic 'Shift' and 'Drift'

Variations in circulating influenza types, subtypes, and strain types are responsible for the characteristic epidemiologic patterns of recurring infection and disease associated with influenza. Influenza viruses undergo two distinct forms of antigenic variation. Antigenic shift occurs infrequently and reflects the appearance of influenza strains with surface glycoproteins that are antigenically dissimilar to previous strains; this is recognized only with type A viruses. There is low homology between the new HA and the previous one. In shift, the HA always changes; the NA may or may not. Shift is recognized by the subtype description in the identification of type A viruses. Pandemics usually follow after shift has occurred.

In contrast, antigenic drift occurs routinely and reflects minor antigenic changes in either or both of the surface glycoproteins. It occurs with all three influenza types, but has been studied most extensively in types A and B. It is responsible for the need to update the vaccine regularly.

The mechanism responsible for shift is a result of the fact that influenza viruses exhibit a high frequency of genetic reassortment because of their segmented genome. Influenza viruses of the same type but with different genetic properties may simultaneously infect cells. During the virion assembly process, gene segments from either parent virus may be included in progeny virions that may then exhibit characteristics of either parent. Among influenza A viruses, antigenic shift or emergence of new subtypes is thought to be the result of this genetic reassortment. In addition, influenza A subtypes infecting non-human species (birds and swine) provide a gene pool for new human subtypes. These new subtypes in nonhuman species probably develop as a result of reassortment and mutation, and subsequent animal-human contact could initiate infection in the human population. Antigenic shifts and the resulting introduction of influenza variants to a large, susceptible population result in pandemic situations, with high attack rates and increased morbidity and mortality. An example of reassortment that resulted in a major pandemic, apparently occurred in 1957. Five gene segments of the new human virus A(H2N2) came from the previous human strain. However, three gene segments most probably came from an avian strain. These were the segments coding for PB1, HA, and NA. With a new HA and NA, a pandemic resulted.

In contrast to the major genetic changes contributed by antigenic shift, minor antigenic changes in the HA and NA surface glycoproteins of influenza A and B occur sequentially with time, resulting in antigenic drift. These progressive changes may sometimes involve only a single amino acid change if they are in the appropriate region, but they usually involve more. They alter the antigenic characteristics of HA and NA in such a way that neutralizing antibodies produced as a result of previous infection or vaccination provide little or no protection. These mutations are likely to emerge as a result of selection of variants that are less susceptible to neutralizing antibodies present in the population. In terms of contemporary viruses, drift occurs most rapidly with the A(H3N2) viruses, and they must be replaced most often in the vaccine. If antigenic drift occurs between the time that the vaccine is formulated and the time that it is administered, its effectiveness would be reduced. To reduce the likelihood of this happening, continual influenza surveillance with antigenic characterization of isolates and annual reformulation of vaccines are required. An exception to the historic view that reassortment alone can produce a pandemic virus has now been documented in the reconstructed 1918 virus. As described in detail in Chapter 15, this virus, whose RNA was recovered from human tissues only recently, is fully avian in origin. It is not a combined human-avian reassortment, but rather a humanized avian virus, so that it can attack and replicate in humans. Its virulence has been shown to be related not to just the gene coding for the hemagglutinin, but to several of the genes interacting.

Summary

Influenza types A, B, and C are three antigenically distinct genera within the family of orthomyxoviruses. Type A and B viruses infect the human respiratory tract, with resulting production of progeny virions and generation of symptoms to guarantee spread of virus to susceptible hosts.

Both type A and B influenza viruses undergo antigenic variation defined as drift (minor changes). These changes are a result of point mutations in the HA and NA of the virus. They occur continuously, and, as a result, vaccines need to be updated regularly. Major changes, referred to as shift, occur only with type A viruses. They are a result of reassortment, a situation in which, following coinfection, gene segments of another virus replace segments in the prior human virus. The result is a new type A subtype and, typically, pandemic spread. The 1918 virus is an exception to this rule.

Antibodies to HA and NA protect, and production of these antibodies is the purpose of vaccination. The functions of the M2 protein of type A virus and the NA of type A and B viruses are the targets of current antivirals. Other activities of the virus may become future targets.

Suggested Readings

Cox NJ, Kawaoka Y: Orthomyxoviruses: influenza. In: Collier L, Balows A, Sussman M, eds. *Topley & Wilson's Microbiology and Microbial Infections, Vol 1: Virology*, 9th ed. London, Edward Arnold, pp 385-433, 1997.

Cox NJ, Subbarao K: Influenza. *Lancet* 1999;354:1277-1282.

Nicholson KG, Webster RG, Hay AJ, eds. *Textbook of Influenza*. Oxford, Blackwell Science Ltd, 1998.

Chapter 4

Immunology and Pathogenesis

Pathogenesis of Influenza Infection

Influenza is transmitted from an infected person to a susceptible person by airborne spread or, less frequently, by direct contact. The susceptible person inhales small, airborne particles of virus-containing respiratory secretions that are released when an infected person coughs or sneezes. The fact that the lower respiratory tract is typically involved in the infection supports this understanding of the method of transmission, as does the rapid increase in disease occurrence in the community. Data from experimental human infections suggest that the dose required to initiate infection in the lower respiratory tract is much lower than that required in the nasopharynx.

Infection begins in the tracheobronchial epithelium when the virus attacks respiratory columnar epithelial cells; it is likely that the entire respiratory tract can be infected by the influenza virus. Cellular infection is initiated by attachment of viral hemagglutinin (HA) to cell surface receptors that contain N-acetylneuraminic acid (sialic acid). The mucous layer covering the respiratory epithelium contains mucoproteins with sialic acid residues. Viral neuraminidase (NA) plays an active role in promoting cellular infection by facilitating viral penetration through respiratory secretions. Following its attachment to a respiratory epithelial cell, the virus enters the cell, is uncoated, and releases viral ribonucleoprotein into the cellular cytoplasm. Transcription and replication of the viral genome take place in the nucleus of the virus-infected cell, followed by synthesis of viral proteins and replication of viral RNA. The virus is assembled at the cell surface, with budding of progeny virions at sites altered by the insertion of viral HA and NA. As the progeny virions are released into extracellular fluid, they infect adjacent epithelial cells and have the potential to spread to large areas of the respiratory tract. The incubation period from exposure to onset of virus shedding and illness is 1 to 5 days; virus shedding may be detected before illness onset. The duration of virus shedding is 3 to 5 days in adults; it is longer in children and immunocompromised persons.

Host cells infected with the influenza virus ultimately undergo cell death (apoptosis) as their protein synthesis is inhibited. Virus-infected cells shed virus for about 8 hours before ceasing metabolic activity; dying cells are sloughed off into the lumen of the respiratory tract. As cellular infection progresses, the respiratory epithelium may be denuded down to the basement membrane, with significant disruption of normal ciliary activity. This loss of respiratory epithelial cells contributes to symptomatic illness with impairment of pulmonary function and tracheobronchial clearance. Infection initiates host defense mechanisms that lead to mucosal inflammation and edema; infiltration of polymorphonuclear cells, lymphocytes, and macrophages into the respiratory mucosa; activation of the humoral and cell-mediated immune responses; and production of cytokines. Although these processes lead to illness resolution, they also contribute to the development of illness symptoms. Production of proinflammatory cytokines, which is an attempt by the body to fight off the infection, becomes part of the mechanism that produces the influenza syndrome and has been identified as a possible explanation of systemic features of influenza infection. Complications of influenza infection may include primary viral pneumonia characterized by alveolar edema, cellular

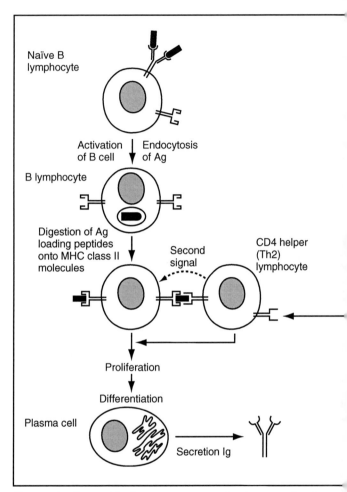

Figure 1: A simplified representation of induction of a B lymphocyte (antibody) response, showing the major cell types involved. (1) A naïve B lymphocyte binds a protein antigen via its surface immunoglobulin (Ig), which recognizes a specific epitope on the protein. This protein is then endocytosed and processed through the exogenous major histocompatibility

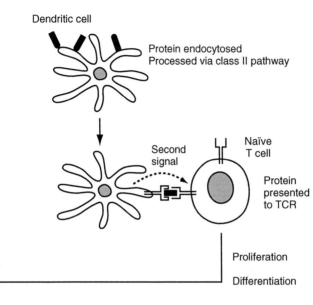

Dendritic cell

Protein endocytosed
Processed via class II pathway

Second signal

Naïve T cell

Protein presented to TCR

Proliferation

Differentiation

Key:

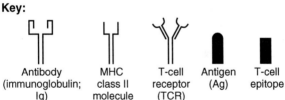

| Antibody (immunoglobulin; Ig) | MHC class II molecule | T-cell receptor (TCR) | Antigen (Ag) | T-cell epitope |

complex (MHC) class II pathway, and the B cell presents (on its surface) a peptide (different from the epitope that binds to the Ig molecules on its surface) bound to its class II molecules. (2) Dendritic cells endocytose the protein, process it through the class II pathway, and present peptides bound to MHC class II molecules.

(caption continued on next page)

infiltrates, and fibrosis. Altered mucociliary clearance may also allow secondary invasion by pathogenic bacteria that colonize the nasopharynx and cause pneumonia, sinusitis, and otitis media. The entire respiratory tract may become infected, and the reparative process may take many weeks to completely resolve the injury. Avian infection in humans is a possible exception to the general rule that influenza is limited to the respiratory tract. This system is further discussed in Chapter 15.

Immune Response to Influenza Infection

Recovery from influenza infection and protection against reinfection are associated with specific host immune responses. Influenza infection induces a cascade of nonspecific and specific host immune responses that involve complement, alveolar macrophages, natural killer (NK) cells, $CD8^+$ cytolytic T (Tc) and $CD4^+$ helper T (Th) lymphocytes, neutralizing antibodies (B lymphocytes/plasma cells), and cytokines (eg, interferon). Nonspecific inhibition of influenza infection may occur early in infection and includes increased interferon levels, which

---

Figure 1: *(caption continued from previous page)* The peptides are recognized by a subset of naïve CD4 T lymphocytes bearing the cognate T-cell receptors, which then proliferate, differentiate, and act as helper cells (CD4 Th2 cells). (3) CD4 Th2 cells recognize the peptides presented by B cells on their class II MHC molecules and stimulate B cells in two ways. First, CD4 cells provide a second signal via the CD40-CD40 ligand pathway; CD40 ligand on CD4 cells binds CD40 on B cells, initiating B-cell intracellular signaling. Second, CD4 cells secrete cytokines (IL-4, IL-10) that stimulate the presenting B lymphocytes to proliferate and differentiate into end-stage plasma cells that secrete their epitope-specific Ig molecules. Reprinted with permission from Nathanson N, Ahmed R, Brinton MA, et al: *Viral Pathogenesis and Immunity.* Philadelphia: Lippincott Williams & Wilkins, 2001:59.

inhibit viral replication and stimulate the immune response, complement-mediated lysis, increased NK cell activity, and virus inhibition by various mucins and lectins in respiratory secretions. Cytokines are produced by influenza-infected cells and by cells participating in the immune response; they have antiviral properties and regulate the immune response. Specific immune responses include the activation of $CD8^+$ Tc cells to eliminate virus-infected cells and the production of specific antibody for neutralization of free virions before more cells are infected. $CD4^+$ Th cells coordinate the specific antibody response, which is carried out by B lymphocytes. $CD8^+$ Tc cell activity and the $CD4^+$ Th cell-dependent antibody response play significant roles in recovery from an established influenza infection. Specific T and B lymphocyte clones are directed at antigenic sites (epitopes) on the internal influenza proteins NP and M1 and at sites on HA and NA surface proteins.

Humoral Immunity

The humoral immune response to influenza infection involves the synthesis of antibodies to viral proteins, including the HA, NA, NP and M1 proteins. The humoral immune response is activated as B lymphocytes bind viral protein antigen via a surface immunoglobulin that recognizes a specific epitope on the viral protein and present processed antigen on their surface in association with major histocompatibility complex (MHC) class II molecules. Likewise, specifically differentiated $CD4^+$ Th (Th2) cells recognize viral antigens presented with MHC class II molecules on activated B lymphocytes. Through a signaling process and secretion of cytokines, $CD4^+$ Th cells induce these activated B lymphocytes to proliferate and differentiate into plasma cells capable of secreting epitope-specific immunoglobulin (antibody). This process is shown in Figure 1. The antibody formed represents all major immunoglobulin classes, IgM, IgG, and IgA. The early response to infection is characterized by IgM immunoglobulins; IgG and IgA, including secretory IgA that is active in the respiratory tract, appear later in infection and characterize the response to reinfection.

Antibodies produced in response to antigenic stimulation act in the host's defense in several ways. Neutralizing antibodies, which are usually directed against major antigenic sites on the viral HA, can bind to the virus and neutralize infectivity by preventing the virus' attachment to host cell receptors. This form of antibody-mediated protection is limited to antigenically related viral subtypes. Non-neutralizing antibodies directed against other viral antigens may interfere with later steps in viral entry into host cells. Virions bound to immunoglobulins are readily phagocytosed and destroyed by macrophages in a process known as opsonization. Antibodies can also interact with NK cells that then carry out antibody-dependent, cell-mediated, cytotoxic attacks on virus-infected cells.

Antibody to HA is induced by the inactivated vaccine used today. Protection from infection in healthy adults has been associated with an HA antibody titer of 1:40. This titer is commonly mentioned in regulatory requirements of the European Union.

Cell-Mediated Immunity

The cell-mediated immune response begins with binding and processing of viral antigen by antigen-presenting cells, dendritic cells, and macrophages, which express MHC class I and II molecules. CD8+ Tc cells are effector cells that are signaled to proliferate and differentiate when they recognize viral antigens (proteolytically cleaved virion fragments) presented by the antigen-presenting cells in association with MHC class I molecules. CD4+ Th (Th1) cells assist the CD8+ Tc cell response through production of cytokines (IFN-γ and IL-2). This process is shown in Figure 2. CD8+ Tc cells are cytolytic to target cells (influenza-infected respiratory cells) carrying the viral antigen that induced their proliferation, and they produce cytokines to attract inflammatory cells for the elimination of virus and dead host cells. CD4$^+$ Th cells also recognize viral antigen presented by antigen-presenting cells, but in association with MHC class II molecules; CD4$^+$ Th cells differentiate and proliferate before they interact with activated B lymphocytes in the humoral immune response as described above.

Antigen-specific CD8$^+$ Tc cells are the key effectors of virus clearance and operate primarily by perforin-mediated, contact-dependent cell lysis. Perforin molecules produce channels in the plasma membranes of target cells, which leads to cell lysis. CD8$^+$ Tc cells also secrete serine esterases that enter the target cells and trigger apoptosis before new virions are produced or released. CD8$^+$ Tc cells are not damaged by this process and can destroy multiple target cells. The cell-mediated immune response, unlike the specific antibody response, may provide cross-reactive protection between distinct virus subtypes because T cells recognize the conserved influenza internal proteins (M1 or NP). Live vaccines activate the cell-mediated immune response and the humoral response (production of antibodies); current inactivated vaccines do not. This is considered a possible advantage of the live vaccine approach.

Cytokines

Cytokines, including various interferons (IFN-α, IFN-β, and IFN-γ), interleukins (IL-1, IL-2, IL-4, and IL-6), and tumor necrosis factor (TNF-α), are produced by virus-infected cells and by lymphocytes (CD4$^+$ Th and CD8$^+$ Tc cells) participating in the immune response. Cytokines have antiviral properties and regulate the immune response; however, they may also contribute to the symptoms and pathology associated with influenza infection. Cytokine functions are complex, with synergistic and antagonistic roles. The interferons and IL-2 are thought to have protective roles, while IL-1, IL-6, and TNF-α are involved in the inflammatory response and production of symptoms

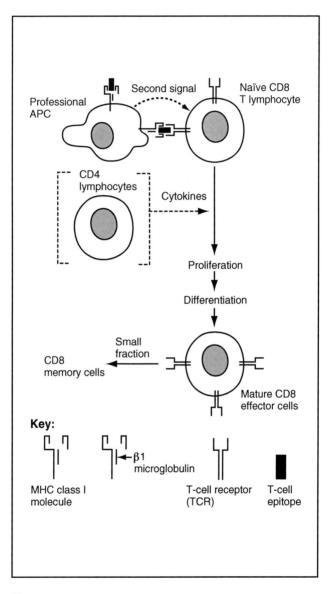

Professional APC

Second signal

Naïve CD8 T lymphocyte

CD4 lymphocytes

Cytokines

Proliferation

Differentiation

Small fraction

CD8 memory cells

Mature CD8 effector cells

Key:

MHC class I molecule

←β1 microglobulin

T-cell receptor (TCR)

T-cell epitope

in addition to their protective roles. IFN-α may also have a role in symptom production. The interferons induce an antiviral state in cells and regulate the immune response by stimulation of macrophages and NK cell activity, control of immunoglobulin class switching and antibody production, and up-regulation of MHC expression. IL-2 is a key factor in the cell-mediated response because it stimulates the clonal expansion of CD8$^+$ cells; IL-4 drives the clonal expansion of B cells.

Cytokine proinflammatory functions contribute to the systemic features of influenza infection. IL-1 can induce fever, sleep, anorexia, and hypotension. TNF-α produces fever and anorexia as part of its proinflammatory role; however, it also has beneficial cytotoxic functions.

Figure 2: A simplified representation of induction of a cellular immune response showing the major cell types involved. A professional antigen-presenting cell (APC) bears major histocompatibility complex (MHC) class I molecules that present a specific peptide bound to the antigen-binding groove. Naïve CD8 T lymphocytes expressing a T-cell receptor that recognizes the same peptide will bind to the peptide and be stimulated to proliferate. Proliferation is triggered by two 'signals': the recognition of the peptide and cross-linking of interactive accessory proteins on the surfaces of APCs and naïve T cells (such as CD40-CD40 ligand). The ability to provide this second signal distinguishes professional APCs from most other cells that express class I molecules. Following proliferation, CD8 lymphocytes differentiate into mature CD8 T lymphocytes that are capable of recognizing and 'killing' target cells bearing the same epitope on their class I molecules. For many viruses, CD4 helper T lymphocytes (via cytokines such as IL-2 and IL-4) and activated dendritic cells appear to play a limited role in induction of CD8 responses. CD8 memory cells are likely derived from the CD8 effector cell pool. Reprinted with permission from Nathanson N, Ahmed R, Brinton MA, et al: *Viral Pathogenesis and Immunity*. Philadelphia: Lippincott Williams & Wilkins, 2001:60.

IL-6 is involved in T- and B-cell activation and differentiation and is a potent fever inducer. Other cytokines and active agents, including chemokines, also have roles in host defense that are critical to resolution of disease but that may be expressed as symptoms. Symptomatic relief through management of proinflammatory cytokines would seem desirable. However, separation of cytokine symptom roles from those roles essential to resolution of influenza infection may be difficult. The fact that antivirals reduce the need for antipyretics, for example, shows that directly attacking viral replication reduces symptoms mediated by cytokine responses. Dysregulation of the immune response may occur with aging and other conditions and may include a change in cytokine balance, with increased production of proinflammatory cytokines.

Mechanisms of Prevention and Recovery

The various host defenses change in importance according to whether they are involved in recovery from primary influenza infection or in prevention of or recovery from reinfection. During primary infection, the cell-mediated immune response can react quickly with large numbers of CD8+ Tc effector cells that destroy virus-infected cells; the antibody response develops more slowly and acts most efficiently on infectious virus before cellular infection. Therefore, the cell-mediated response is most critical to host defense during primary infection.

Previous infection induces a temporary immune state and may provide protection from reinfection, from clinically apparent influenza illness, or from the serious complications of infection. Significant titers of specific antiviral antibodies are maintained in the immune host for periods following primary infection. These antibodies are in the circulation (IgG) and mucosal fluids (secretory IgA) and are available to immediately neutralize influenza viruses and prevent cellular infection. Immunity from reinfection correlates with significant titers of mucosal antibody (secretory IgA). Reexposure induces an anamnestic response with higher antibody titers, as well as greater biological activity of antibody against specific influenza antigens. The immune host also maintains memory CD4$^+$ Th and CD8$^+$ Tc cells that, on reexposure to specific influenza antigen, proliferate rapidly to contain the infection; these cells may respond to a lower threshold of antigen stimulation than unprimed cells. Maintenance of T memory cells in a stable state of readiness may be managed by cytokines. Because the cell-mediated and humoral immune responses to influenza exposure are antigen specific, protection is limited. Antibodies, the first line of defense, are typically directed to antigenic sites on the HA glycoprotein; therefore, they afford no protection against exposure to an unrelated influenza type or subtype (antigenic shift) and only limited efficacy in the event of significant antigenic drift.

The immune response to the trivalent inactivated vaccine is imperfect because it is characterized by systemic increases in specific IgG antibodies to influenza HA of the various component strains, but it initiates little protective mucosal response. As a result, the primary benefit of vaccination is in protecting recipients, especially older persons, from serious illness or complications of influenza infection rather than from infection and illness. Vaccine effectiveness is also limited by the variation of circulating strains from those strains included in the vaccine. The live-attenuated vaccine in development is likely to offer better protection because its nature and route of administration mimic those of natural infection, and the immune response to it is likely to be improved and include mucosal protection.

Summary

The cell-mediated immune response, characterized by cytolytic T-cell destruction of virus-infected cells, and the humoral immune response, characterized by helper T cell dependent antibody response, play significant roles in recovery from an established influenza infection.

These specific immune responses are assisted by multiple nonspecific host defenses. The major defense against influenza infection is mediated by neutralizing antibodies primarily directed against the viral HA. These antibodies develop in response to previous infection or vaccination; their protective efficacy is limited in the event of antigenic shift or significant antigenic drift. Epidemiologic evidence suggests that immunity that develops following infection is relatively long lasting and may provide protection from reinfection or from clinically apparent or complicated illness with identical or closely related influenza virus strains.

Suggested Readings

Doherty PC, Topham DJ, Tripp RA, et al: Effector CD4+ and CD8+ T-cell mechanisms in the control of respiratory virus infections. *Immunol Rev* 1997;159:105-117.

Fritz RS, Hayden FG, Calfee DP, et al: Nasal cytokine and chemokine responses in experimental influenza A virus infection: results of a placebo-controlled trial of intravenous zanamivir treatment. *J Infect Dis* 1999;180:586-593.

Gerhard W: The role of the antibody response in influenza virus infection. *Curr Top Microbiol Immunol* 2001;260:171-190.

Han SN, Meydani SN: Antioxidants, cytokines, and influenza infection in aged mice and elderly humans. *J Infect Dis* 2000; 182(suppl):S74-S80.

Hayden FG, Fritz R, Lobo MC, et al: Local and systemic cytokine responses during experimental human influenza A virus infection. Relation to symptom formation and host defense. *J Clin Invest* 1998;101:643-649.

Nathanson N, Ahmed R, Brinton MA, et al: *Viral Pathogenesis and Immunity*. Philadelphia: Lippincott Williams & Wilkins, 2002.

Zambon MC. The pathogenesis of influenza in humans. *Rev Med Virol* 2001;11:227-241.

Chapter 5

Disease and Complications

Influenza has been described as an unchanging disease caused by a changing virus. This refers to the fact that the type A viruses may undergo shift and drift, and the type B viruses may undergo drift, but the disease described in the 1940s is similar to that observed today, at least in terms of the general characteristics of influenza illness in an individual patient. However, when the influenza illnesses seen today are aggregated by type or subtype, distinct differences in characteristics are apparent. Type A(H3N2) disease is the most severe, and type A(H1N1) disease is the most mild; type B disease is intermediate.[1] Disease characteristics also vary with patient age. Characteristics of influenza produced in humans by the A(H5N1) avian virus are described in Chapter 15.

Classic Influenza Syndrome

Kilbourne created a summary of symptoms reported in a number of early studies. As shown in Table 1, the characteristics of symptoms associated with type A and B viruses are generally similar. Of particular note is the high frequency of cough and fever, a constant finding. The incubation period, or time from virus transmission to development of symptoms, is 1 to 4 days, although it can be longer; some epidemiologic studies have suggested an incubation period of up to 6 days. Onset of illness is sudden, and the symptoms often increase rapidly in severity.

Table 1: Frequency of Signs and Symptoms of Influenza in Older Children and Adults

Sign or Symptom	Frequency	
	Type A Illness	*Type B Illness*
Cough, fever	90%	90%
Headache	80%	60%
Sudden onset, pharyngeal injection	70%	—
Myalgia, conjunctival injection	60%	50%
Sore throat	50%	70%
Substernal pain	40%	—
Anorexia	—	30%

Kilbourne ED: *Influenza.* New York: Plenum Medical Book Company, 1987.

Patients often can report exactly when they began to feel sick. The earliest symptoms include headache and shivering, but cough and discomfort in breathing are sometimes seen. Thereafter, profound prostration and muscular aching begin, along with nasal congestion or discharge. The face is flushed, and there is often conjunctival injection. Sore throat is rarely an early prominent symptom. Temperature rises rapidly to a peak and may remain high for up to 72 hours. Cough, usually dry and often painful, may occasionally be delayed but is one of the most frequently reported symptoms. Gastrointestinal symptoms may occur but are not prominent components of the illness.[2]

The above description of a febrile respiratory disease is the basis of the clinical concept of influenza in adults and older children. The pediatric and geriatric concepts have been slower in developing. In fact, recognition of the importance of influenza in very young children is a relatively recent development. Fever is often higher in children than in adults, and gastrointestinal manifestations such as diarrhea and abdominal pain are more common. Absence of respiratory symptoms is rare.[3] Febrile convulsions sometimes occur. Type A influenza is a recognized cause of croup and, sometimes, bronchitis.[4] One study showed that 14% of children hospitalized with croup actually had influenza. The reason influenza has sometimes not been recognized in young children is not that the illness is so different from that seen in older children but rather that febrile respiratory illnesses of other causes are common in this age group. The index of suspicion should be high when influenza is known to be in the community and the typical illness is seen in older children. In infants, influenza may be harder to identify clinically, but it should be remembered during known periods of transmission. Influenza has been reported out of season among infants in intensive care settings. The availability of antivirals increases the importance of making an appropriate diagnosis. Frail elderly in nursing homes also may not exhibit the typical febrile influenza syndrome, although they may go on to develop life-threatening complications such as pneumonia. Independently living older adults usually exhibit the typical illness, albeit with less fever.

Even in adults and older children, not all cases of influenza fit the description of the typical febrile influenza syndrome. Estimates vary, but some studies suggest that while 70% to 80% of illnesses of influenza etiology are febrile in younger children, the percentage is closer to 50% to 60% in adults. About half of recognized influenza illnesses result in physician consultations, and bed disability is more common with influenza than any other common respiratory infection.[5] The difference in severity by influenza type can be characterized by illness duration in adults; the average time until all symptoms cease is 15 days for type A(H3N2), 13 days for type B, and 10 days for type A(H1N1). Likewise, complications are most likely to develop with A(H3N2) illness and least likely to develop with A(H1N1). Risk groups (ie, persons who are more likely to develop complications because of underlying conditions) are listed in Chapter 6.

Complications of Influenza

There are countless reports of various morbid conditions either accompanying or following influenza infection. Table 2 lists those reported most often. Acute bronchitis may be considered another manifestation of influenza, given influenza's primary manifestation as tracheobronchitis. However, following the febrile episode, cough with sputum production may continue. Acute bronchitis following influenza varies in frequency, but it is considered the most common observed complication. Antibiotics are frequently prescribed for this condition, but results are variable because the illness is often not of bacterial origin. Use of neuraminidase inhibitors for treatment of the primary infection may reduce the likelihood of development of acute bronchitis.

Otitis media has traditionally been considered to be of bacterial etiology, which would justify the use of antibiotics in treatment. However, it is well known that otitis media follows different respiratory infections, and it was hypothesized that viruses provided the initial insult, either by direct infection or by blocking the eustachian tubes and allowing invasion of colonizing bacteria, especially *Streptococcus pneumoniae.* With the advent of polymerase chain reaction (PCR) technology, it became possible to demonstrate the presence of viral nucleic acid in middle ear fluid. The most convincing data on the frequency of otitis media as a complication of influenza have come from recent vaccine and antiviral studies that suggest that

Table 2: Complications of Influenza

Common, Less Severe

- Otitis media in children
- Acute bronchitis
- Exacerbation of asthma in children and adults
- Exacerbation of chronic obstructive pulmonary disease
- Myositis

Uncommon, More Severe

- Pneumonia
  – Primary viral
  – Secondary bacterial
- Cardiovascular complications
- Myocarditis and pericarditis
- Encephalopathy
- Reye's syndrome

approximately 40% of otitis media cases in the influenza season are caused by influenza. Primary prophylaxis with vaccine or treatment with antivirals can prevent the development of otitis media.[6,7]

Exacerbations of Asthma and COPD

As with otitis media, acute respiratory infections have long been recognized to be precipitants of asthma and chronic obstructive pulmonary disease (COPD). Asthma is by far the most common chronic respiratory condition of children, so asthmatic attacks are one of the most common complications of influenza in this group. Other agents, such as the rhinoviruses, may cause more illnesses or asthmatic episodes, but influenza can produce a more severe primary syndrome. The overall effects of the episode may be substantial, with the possibility that more uncommon lower respiratory complications may follow. As a result, vaccine is recommended to prevent the entire asthma episode.[8]

Until recently, the relationship between viral infection and asthma in adults was more difficult to establish than that between viral infection and childhood asthma. PCR techniques have confirmed that while bacterial infection precipitates asthma more frequently in adults than in children, viral infections are also common precipitants of asthma in adults. Influenza has been documented to cause severe exacerbations of asthma in adults, including status asthmaticus.[9] Examination of national data has resulted in reported increases in deaths from influenza among asthmatics; these deaths are probably caused by more common lower respiratory complications, some of which may be bacterial.

Much of the data on asthma in adults and those with COPD are from studies performed in the United Kingdom that associated influenza not only with exacerbations, but also with more severe complications and death. The severity of the complications was related to the severity of the underlying condition. Recent studies have also confirmed that patients with markedly reduced forced expiratory volume in 1 second have difficulty in absorbing the insult of even a mild respiratory infection.

Myositis

While myalgia is a typical symptom of clinical influenza, some influenza outbreaks have been marked by frequent reports of true myositis or even rhabdomyolysis. These reports are most common in type B outbreaks. Clinically, pain is localized in the gastrocnemius and soleus muscles and causes difficulty in walking. This syndrome is more commonly observed in children. In older individuals, there may be signs of rhabdomyolysis, with elevated creatine phosphokinase values.[10]

Pneumonia

The defining complication of influenza is pneumonia, which can be viral, bacterial, or combined. The distinction, which is not always clear, has implications for treatment. Primary viral pneumonia is generally earlier in onset and is often a part of the initial febrile episode. Reports of its frequency and characteristics have varied in past pandemics and in more recent interpandemic influenza. In the 1918 pandemic, lethality was frequently associated with primary influenza pneumonia, which started just 1 or 2 days after the febrile illness began. On autopsy, the lungs were dark and airless, with thin hemorrhagic exudate and no pus. This clearly distinguished the primary pneumonia from another syndrome with evidence of bronchopneumonia that occurred later in onset and, generally, following a period of defervescence. In the 1957 pandemic, primary viral pneumonia was also prominent, especially in those with rheumatic heart disease and particularly in those with mitral stenosis. This pneumonia was associated with congestive heart failure and pulmonary edema. Such observations were not repeated in the 1968 pandemic, perhaps because rheumatic heart disease had become less common in the population.

In general, primary influenza pneumonia should be considered when what appears clinically to be nonbacterial disease without consolidation or segmental involvement begins early in the course of the influenza syndrome. The prognosis of these cases has been poor, and there are little data on improvements resulting from recent advances in intensive care. It is estimated that 80% of primary influenza pneumonia is associated with type A virus; cases associated with type B virus are generally of lower severity.

Secondary Bacterial Pneumonia

Secondary bacterial pneumonia is a more common pulmonary complication of acute influenza. Classically, it presents as a return of fever around day 5, with clinical signs and symptoms of bronchopneumonia. It is thought

Table 3: Bacteria Frequently Involved in Postinfluenza Pneumonia*

- *Streptococcus pneumoniae*
- *Staphylococcus aureus*
- *Haemophilus influenzae*
- Streptococci
- *Klebsiella pneumoniae*
- *Pseudomonas* spp

*Bacteria are listed in order of decreasing frequency of involvement.

that bacteria invade the 'tracheal wound' produced by the influenza virus, which denudes the ciliary epithelium. Lobar and lobular involvement can usually be seen on radiographs. Treatment then requires the selection of the appropriate antibiotic for the bacterial agent involved.

The bacteria that cause pneumonia secondary to influenza infection have changed over time. While the virus causing the 1918 pandemic could not be initially identified, the bacteria could, and *Haemophilus influenzae* influenza was identified more commonly than in more recent epidemics. In the 1957 pandemic, *Staphylococcus aureus* was observed most commonly in hospitalized patients; there are suggestions that this was a result of the higher severity of illness caused by this agent, and that *S pneumoniae* predominated overall. The emergence of antibiotic-resistant *S aureus* may have contributed to these observations[11]; in autopsy series involving type A and B viruses, *S aureus* is the most common single agent. Table 3 lists bacteria that are typically involved in pneumonia secondary to influenza infection in descending order of frequency.

There are many reports of mixed pneumonia infections, which are difficult to interpret and may involve specimen-collecting techniques likely to be contaminated by colonizing bacteria. Antibiotic treatment has not clearly produced a decline in mortality in hospitalized cases of mixed pneumonia. Again, this may be because only patients with the most severe and complicated illness are hospitalized, and these patients may be more likely to have risk factors such as advanced age and underlying disease. Use of influenza and pneumococcal vaccines to prevent complications is preferable to reliance on antibiotic treatment in these situations. The emergence of antibiotic-resistant pneumococci must also be considered.

Cardiovascular Complications

Even in the 1889-1890 pandemic, there were reports of sharp increases in death from a variety of cardiovascular conditions, including congestive heart failure. Whether these deaths were directly caused by influenza illness or were the result of stress put on the cardiovascular system by other effects of influenza is unclear. Recent data have confirmed that cardiovascular deaths increase in influenza outbreaks and that vaccine may prevent several adverse events related to the cardiovascular system, ranging from myocardial infarction to stroke.

While myocarditis and pericarditis may be less frequent cardiovascular complications, they have been the subject of many reports, including pathologic observations from autopsies. The 1957 pandemic resulted in many case series, with reports of arrhythmia, cardiomyopathy, and restrictive myopathy. Electrocardiogram abnormalities were observed in many hospitalized individuals. With the development of cardiospecific isoenzyme testing, the direct effect of the infection on the myocardium could be confirmed. The high frequency of elevated cardiac isoenzymes compared to the low frequency of symptoms suggests that myopathies are common but are mainly asymptomatic.[12]

Pericarditis has rarely been reported after the 1918 pandemic. Occasional case reports have included effusion and constrictive pericarditis. The pathogenesis of myocarditis and pericarditis is not clear. There have been very few reports of isolation of virus from tissue, and it is thought that influenza rarely results in viremia.

Encephalitis and Encephalopathy

Because reports of central nervous system complications are rare, it is difficult to be sure that these complications are related to influenza itself. Cases may be divided into those with normal cerebrospinal fluid (CSF), which could be classified as encephalopathy, and those with abnormal CSF with increases in cells and/or protein abnormalities, which could be classified as encephalitis.[13] Cases with stupor and coma, as well as a variety of other findings such as aphasia, cerebellar ataxia, papilledema, and paresis, including cranial nerve paralysis, have been reported. The interval between the onset of influenza syndrome and the central nervous system complication is between 3 and 8 days. While these complications are uncommon and sometimes of questionable etiology, they are among the most severe, especially in children, in whom they can result in death or long-term disability.[14] There have been occasional reports of isolation of influenza virus or, more recently, influenza RNA from tissue or CSF, but in most cases, any etiologic relationship can only be derived from the timing of illness onset.

Convulsions are associated with influenza in children. They are most commonly febrile and usually are not related to the development of encephalopathy. However, an exception has been observed recently in Japan, where convulsions appear to be more frequent in young children than in the United States. These convulsions are more often the prodrome of an episode of encephalopathy, which can have lethal consequences, and seem to occur most commonly in A(H3N2) outbreaks. Studies are currently under way to determine if this unusual form of postinflu-enza encephalopathy is related to antipyretic or analgesic drugs commonly used in Japan. Encephalopathy has also been reported recently in the US; whether it is as frequent as in Asia is under study, but initial results suggest that it is not.

Reye's Syndrome

During the 1970s and 1980s, Reye's syndrome, an acute encephalopathy with fatty infiltration of the liver, would have been listed among the more common severe complications of influenza in the United States. Reye's syndrome, first described in 1963, was known to follow influenza and varicella infections and occurred almost exclusively in children younger than 18 years. It came to medical and public attention during the type B outbreaks of 1974, when clusters of cases occurred in many states. The disease was often severe, with a high fatality rate and residual mental retardation. Clinically, it was characterized by acute onset of vomiting, disorientation, combativeness, and, finally, coma. Cerebral edema was a common pathologic feature, and reducing it resulted in improved prognosis. Marked increases in liver enzymes were characteristic, and there were pathognomic changes on liver biopsy. However, because liver biopsy results could not be used for epidemiologic studies, the characteristic finding that distinguished the syndrome was elevated blood ammonia, one of the elements of the Centers for Disease Control and Prevention (CDC) case definition. The full definition was (1) acute encephalopathy with few cells in the CSF, or demonstration of cerebral edema; (2) hepatic involvement with ALT, AST, or serum ammonia three times above normal without significant bilirubinemia; and (3) no other reasonable explanation for the condition, including inborn errors of metabolism.

A few small case-control studies indicated that taking aspirin was the main risk factor for developing the syndrome. However, these studies were criticized for flaws in their design. Finally, a large study with direct CDC involvement was launched. The pilot was so dramatic in demonstrating the role of aspirin as the prime risk factor that the results were published rapidly in the *New England Journal of Medicine* in 1985.[15] As a result, aspirin use for children almost totally stopped; in fact, it was already decreasing, with younger parents more likely to use acetaminophen. Thereafter, the incidence of Reye's syndrome in the United States dropped rapidly; this drop did not occur as completely in other countries. Now, if a Reye's-like case is encountered, it is important to rule out inborn errors of metabolism, as well as various intoxications.[16] The virtual disappearance of a condition as a result of changes in medication prescribing is rare.

Clinical Predictors of Influenza

As indicated previously, the influenza syndrome is characteristic enough that it is usually possible to predict with reasonable certainty that a case under clinical observation is influenza. Several studies have pointed out that fever and cough are the most reliable predictors of influenza infection. Other symptoms, such as chills, myalgia, and nasal congestion, may be common in influenza, but they are also common in noninfluenza illness. Gastrointestinal symptoms are negative predictors; that is, their presence indicates that an illness is less likely to be influenza. In some studies, conjunctival injection was more likely in influenza, but because subsequent studies have not recorded the incidence of conjunctival injection, this finding has not been confirmed. A study conducted in France concluded that cough and fever were the most important predictors but that they predicted influenza only about 40% of the time. However, during the influenza season, when influenza is known to be present in the community, this frequency increases to 79% to 87%.[17,18] The utility of influenza predictors, formerly of only scientific interest, is now critical in determining who to treat with influenza antivirals, which is examined in Chapters 13 and 16.

References

1. Monto AS, Koopman JS, Longini IM Jr: Tecumseh study of illness. XIII. Influenza infection and disease, 1976-1981. *Am J Epidemiol* 1985;121:811-822.

2. Kilbourne ED: Influenza in man. In: *Influenza*. New York, Plenum Medical Book Co, 1987.

3. Price DA, Postlethwaite RJ, Longson M: Influenza virus A2 infections presenting with febrile convulsions and gastrointestinal symptoms in young children. *Clin Pediatr* 1976;15:361-367.

4. Kim HW, Brandt CD, Arrobio JO, et al: Influenza A and B virus infection in infants and young children during the years 1957-1976. *Am J Epidemiol* 1979;109:464-479.

5. Monto AS, Kioumehr F: The Tecumseh Study of Respiratory Illness. IX. Occurrence of influenza in the community, 1966-1971. *Am J Epidemiol* 1975;102:553-563.

6. Belshe RB, Mendelman PM, Treanor J, et al: Efficacy of live attenuated, cold-adapted, trivalent, intranasal influenza virus vaccine in children. *N Engl J Med* 1998;338:1405-1412.

7. Whitley RJ, Hayden FG, Reisinger KS, et al: Oral oseltamivir treatment of influenza in children. *Pediatr Infect Dis J* 2001;20:127-133.

8. Minor TE, Dick EC, Baker JW, et al: Rhinovirus and influenza type A infections as precipitants of asthma. *Am Rev Resp Dis* 1976;113:149-153.

9. Nicholson KG, Kent J, Ireland DC: Respiratory viruses and exacerbations of asthma in adults. *BMJ* 1993;307:982-986.

10. Baine WB, Luby JP, Martin SM: Severe illness with influenza B. *Am J Med* 1980;68:181-189.

11. Petersdorf RG, Fusco JJ, Harter DH, et al: Pulmonary infections complicating Asian influenza. *Arch Intern Med* 1959;103:262-272.

12. Proby CM, Hackett D, Gupta S, et al: Acute myopericarditis in influenza A infection. *Q J Med* 1986;60:887-892.

13. Dunbar JM, Jamieson WM, Langlands JH, et al: Encephalitis and influenza. *Br Med J* 1958;i:913-15.

14. Flewett TH, Hoult JG: Influenzal encephalopathy and post-influenzal encephalitis. *Lancet* 1958;2:11-15.

15. Hurwitz ES, Barrett MJ, Bregman D, et al: Public Health Service study on Reye's syndrome and medications. Report of the pilot phase. *N Engl J Med* 1985;313:849-857.

16. Belay ED, Bresee JS, Holman RC, et al: Reye's syndrome in the United States from 1981 through 1997. *N Engl J Med* 1999;340: 1377-1382.

17. Monto AS, Gravenstein S, Elliott M, et al: Clinical signs and symptoms predicting influenza infection. *Arch Intern Med* 2000; 160:3243-3247.

18. Boivin G, Hardy I, Tellier G, et al: Predicting influenza infections during epidemics with use of a clinical case definition. *Clin Infect Dis* 2000;31:1166-1169.

Chapter 6

Epidemiology

Cycling and Seasonality of Influenza

One of the reasons influenza is so recognizable on an individual and an epidemiologic basis is its seasonality. The basic observation that influenza occurs during cold weather applies to the northern and southern temperate zones, except when a new pandemic variant arises. In North America, A(H3N2) outbreaks usually start in late November and December and peak anywhere from late December through February. A(H1N1) and type B outbreaks generally peak later, often in February and March. However, in many years, type B activity lingers well into April and May. In the southern hemisphere, the influenza season is reversed. If this reversal were precise, then little activity would begin before June. However, in many years, there is already considerable activity by the beginning of June. The timing of influenza outbreaks is important for many reasons, but mostly to determine when to administer vaccine. In the United States, inactivated vaccine generally becomes available in September, and most of it is administered in October and November. In 2000-2001, vaccine was delayed, and many people could not be vaccinated until December. Delayed vaccination is not a problem as long as influenza outbreaks do not start before January. With new manufacturers entering the US market, supplies and availability of vaccine are certain to increase.

Seasonality in the tropics is different, with various patterns being reported. In Singapore, on the equator, influenza may be reported in any month, but cases tend to concentrate at specific times, often with a peak of illness. Some areas that have little temperature change year round and a profound dry season have a single major influenza outbreak during the rainy season. This observation presents a paradox: in colder areas, transmission takes place when the humidity is low, while in the tropics, it takes place when the humidity is high. The common factor may be that schools, an important site of transmission, are open in both cases.

For 25 years, two type A influenza virus subtypes and one type B virus have appeared regularly in the human population. Before 1977, when a new A variant appeared, it replaced the previously prevalent one. In 1977, however, the A(H1N1) subtype returned, and both A(H3N2) and A(H1N1) virus continue to circulate. This is likely to be the result of the unusual nature of the reintroduction of the A(H1N1) virus, which was limited to infecting young adults and children who had not been exposed during its previous appearance.[1]

An important question is how often each of the three circulating virus types or subtypes will appear, generally stated as, 'Is next year going to be an A year or a B year?' This is a difficult question to answer because the specifics of influenza occurrence are notoriously unpredictable. One certainty is that every year is an influenza year; however, which viral types will be circulating in a given year cannot be predicted. Therefore, it would be a mistake to examine the last influenza year and to base the use of vaccine in the upcoming year on the patterns observed.

The epidemiologic characteristics of each subtype are much more predictable. Type A viruses occur more frequently than type B viruses; overall, 60% to 80% of isolates obtained over a number of years will be type A. Type A(H3N2) is more common than A(H1N1). At one time, it was thought that A(H1N1) might disappear, after little activity over several seasons. However, in 2000-2001,

A(H1N1) predominated in many parts of the United States, with additional major B activity in some areas. While all three types or subtypes can be isolated somewhere in the United States every year, most local outbreaks are caused by only one or, in some years, two types.

Pandemic Influenza

Occurrence

Even more unpredictable than what the annual incidence of influenza will be and which viruses will be involved is the question of when a pandemic will occur. Pandemics result when type A variants with a new hemagglutinin and, sometimes, a new neuraminidase begin to spread in the human population. The resulting outbreaks are much larger than usual and occur all over the world in a limited period, peaking within months of each other. Influenza pandemics, or what seem to have been influenza pandemics, have been historically tracked. However, the first virologically documented pandemic took place in 1889-1890. This pandemic is thought to have been caused by an H2 virus, but this assumption is based on analysis of collected sera from those who lived through the pandemic and has not been confirmed by direct viral isolation. Serology suggests that in 1900, a variant with new hemagglutinin, H3, emerged, but no pandemic was documented. There is no question about the occurrence of a pandemic in 1918; the dramatic impact of this episode has been the subject of novels as well as scientific writing.[2] The entire genome of the virus that caused it, an A(H1N1) variant, has recently been sequenced from pathologic and other specimens and have been found to be fully avian in origin.[3]

After 1918, as is usual with mammalian influenza viruses, the hemagglutinin and neuraminidase of the type A viruses gradually changed, but no new subtype emerged until 1957. A major antigenic change in 1947 did not result in a new subtype or a pandemic in that year. The 1957 A(H2N2) variant, with new hemagglutinin and neuraminidase, spread around the world rapidly and caused major outbreaks. As is typical in pandemics, these outbreaks occurred out of season, starting in August in the United States. Eleven years later, in 1968, the A(H3N2) virus emerged. Because only the hemagglutinin had changed, the US outbreaks, while large, were not as extreme as in 1957. In Europe, there was not nearly as dramatic an effect on mortality as in the United States. Since 1957, there have been gradual changes in A(H3N2), but this virus has continued to occur for more than 30 years. The reappearance of A(H1N1), described above, might be termed a 'pseudopandemic.' Although global outbreaks occurred in a period of months, they were limited to individuals younger than 25 years.

Mortality

The pattern of mortality seen in pandemic influenza has been documented for more than 100 years. Because of the high incidence of illness and death seen in these episodes, examination of vital records can identify which age groups have been principally affected. Figure 1 shows the mortality reported in Massachusetts in 1892 and the national number of deaths for 1918 and 1957.[4] The 1892 and 1957 pandemics show the pattern of elevated age-specific mortality in very young children, relatively few deaths until approximately age 45, and a sharp increase in deaths at age 65. This is referred to as the 'U' or, more properly, the 'J' shaped curve. The overall death rate was lower in 1957 than in the 19th century pandemic, perhaps because of the availability of antibiotics and other supportive treatments. The U-shaped mortality pattern is also typical of many interpandemic outbreaks.

The exception to the U-shaped pattern can be seen in the 1918 outbreak of Spanish influenza, when there was high mortality in young adults as well as young children and elderly persons. This was a unique occurrence in the history of documented influenza pandemics and is referred

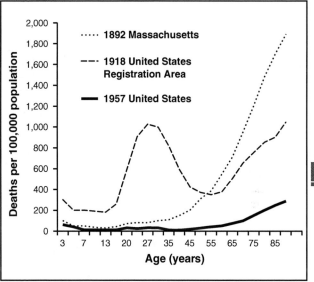

Figure 1: Mortality rates in different influenza pandemics. Dauer et al, *Am Rev Respir Dis* 1961;83:15-28.

to as the 'W' shaped curve. The mortality rate observed in young adults in 1918 was accompanied by clinical descriptions of an illness involving 'heliotrope cyanosis' and pathologic findings of fluid-filled lungs, evidence of primary influenza pneumonia.[5] What is even more striking about the deaths in this age group is that the rates shown in Figure 1 are mortality rates, not case fatality. Case fatality, the proportion of those who are ill that die, would be even higher for young adults than for children, who experienced higher illness rates but lower death rates.

Recent reexamination of mortality data has led to new conclusions about the impact of the 1918 pandemic. The global mortality figure for the 1918 pandemic, originally estimated to be 20 million, has been increased to 40 million or even 60 million. This change was based on the use of

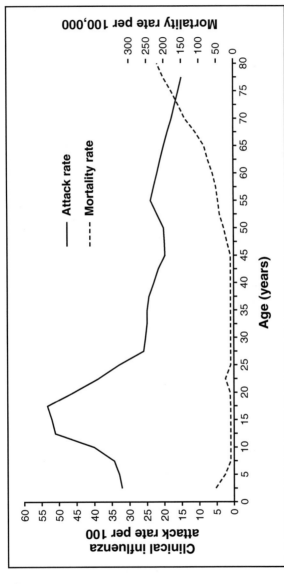

Figure 2: Clinical influenza attack rate (Kansas City, 1957) and annual mortality rate of pneumonia and influenza (United States, 1957). Chin et al, *Public Health Rep* 1960;75:149-158.

modern demographic methods and mainly involved taking into account data from developing countries, which had not been properly counted in the original estimates. In terms of US data, overall life expectancy dipped in 1918, the only time this happened during the 20th century.

In the typical pandemic, such as the one in 1957, excess mortality in healthy adults is not a prominent feature. However, when pandemic mortality by age is compared to interpandemic mortality, it is found that a larger proportion of healthy adults die in a pandemic. In pandemic years, otherwise healthy individuals are at increased risk compared to interpandemic years because they lack immunity to the new strains that are circulating. In interpandemic years, more people have immunity gained through previous exposure to the circulating viruses. Those with underlying conditions are at increased risk in any year.[6]

Morbidity

Since the last true pandemic occurred in 1968-1969, it is difficult to estimate pandemic morbidity using modern techniques. While deaths over the limited period during which the new virus is circulating can be quantified using public records, illnesses cannot. A classic estimation of age-specific morbidity was carried out in the A(H2N2) pandemic of 1957-1958. The method involved use of a case definition without requiring laboratory confirmation of illness etiology. Data on morbidity came from one location, Kansas City.[7] This is shown in Figure 2, along with the mortality rate for the entire United States during the same pandemic. The contrast between the morbidity, which is highest in children and young adults, and the mortality, which is lowest in these age groups, is dramatic. The morbidity reported in this investigation, which reached about 50% in children and 20% to 25% in young adults, indicates the kind of impact this infection had in a general population. Based on recent information, the apparently low morbidity in young children is considered to be an

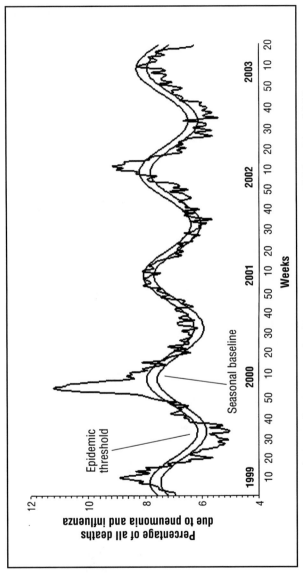

Figure 3: Pneumonia and influenza mortality for 122 US cities, January 1999 to May 2003.

artifact because it is harder to identify disease in this age group using a case definition. Many cases that would be virologically confirmed are not recognized as typical influenza. Regardless of the exact details, illness rates of this magnitude would put a drain on the health-care system because they occur over a short period.

Interpandemic Influenza

Mortality

A method was developed in the early 1960s to track mortality caused by annual influenza outbreaks. It has been reformulated over the years, but it remains the principal way that influenza-related mortality and the overall yearly impact of influenza are quantified.[8,9] Death certificates are examined, and a series of diagnoses that correspond to pneumonia and influenza (P&I) categories are identified and enumerated. Deaths from influenza are usually the result of complicating pneumonias. Other diagnoses, especially those related to cardiovascular disease, could be used to identify influenza-related deaths, but such indicators have been viewed as minimal estimates; that is, they are specific but not very sensitive. The P&I method does not take into account the presence of influenza viruses. In other words, enumeration of P&I deaths does not require virus identification. The P&I deaths from causes other than influenza are then removed from consideration through use of a seasonal baseline, which should be made up of the noninfluenza cases. Cases of P&I in excess of the expected or baseline level are considered to be influenza-related. An epidemiologic threshold is used to take care of random variation. The circulating viruses are identified by an independent surveillance system.

The excess mortality method is used in several ways. The most visible is the rapid tracking of influenza outbreaks. There are 122 cities in the United States that report death diagnosis data to the Centers for Disease Control and Prevention (CDC) on a weekly basis. These data are quickly compiled and are used to assess whether a particular influenza year is severe. An example of the results from the reporting cities is shown in Figure 3. Sustained increases in mortality do not occur every year. The most extreme increases are related to A(H3N2) viruses, although there have been years in which type B virus has caused excess deaths. Excess mortality from type B virus has been rare; excess mortality in years in which A(H1N1) predominates is even more unusual. For example, in 1985-1986, a type B year, P&I deaths were estimated to be 6,700. In the next year, a type A(H1N1) year, this number fell to 1,800.

While P&I mortality is a useful tool in following influenza mortality because of its relative specificity, it misses many deaths that are produced by influenza infection. The total number of deaths during the influenza season has been examined as a way to capture more completely the impact of influenza on mortality. However, this method is not as specific as studying P&I, and it has wider confidence intervals. The relationship of P&I deaths to total deaths can be seen in a severe A(H3N2) year, 1989-1990, when the estimated number of deaths was 10,000 when the P&I outcome was used and 43,600 when the total mortality method was used. From 1979 to 1992, annual influenza-related deaths in the United States ranged from 2,100 to 11,700 according to the P&I method and from 0 to 47,200 according to the total method. A new method that will not have the 'instability' of the total method is under study. This has resulted in the current estimate that 36,000 Americans on the average die each year as a result of influenza. By any standard, the total mortality from influenza is high in most years and requires appropriate action.[10]

Morbidity

Interpandemic influenza morbidity is more difficult to estimate. Typical influenza illness is not difficult to recognize, but many influenza illnesses are of less severity, and many do not occur at the peak of the influenza season; these cases are not usually counted. One of the most comprehensive ways to identify the frequency of influenza infection as opposed to clinical disease is to collect blood samples before and after the influenza season to determine the frequency of rise in antibody titer. A rise in antibody titer is a certain indication that infection has taken place. Figures 4 and 5 show the infection rates with A(H3N2) and type B viruses documented in the community of Tecumseh, Michigan.[11] For A(H3N2) virus, the infection rate is approximately 40% in young children and 15% in adults. For type B virus, the rate in children is approximately the same; the apparent sparing of young children is an artifact, the result of relative insensitivity of the hemagglutinin inhibition test in this age group. In adults, however, the rate is dramatically decreased. Influenza that produces school outbreaks but little illness in adults is probably type B or, possibly, A(H1N1). Major outbreaks in adults and children are likely to be caused by A(H3N2). This probability is increased if there are reports of nursing home outbreaks.

How do the infection rates shown in the figures translate into clinical illness rates? A conservative estimate is that approximately half of infections produce symptomatic disease. Children will probably experience more infections as symptomatic disease than adults because adults are more likely to have been previously exposed to influenza viruses. One common estimate is that the annual influenza attack rate is 10% for adults and 20% for children, but the real rate will differ from year to year based on variations in outbreak severity.[12]

Influenza is the most severe respiratory illness experienced by the general population. Almost 50% of those with influenza illness will consult their physician by telephone or office visit. Influenza illness also produces the highest rates of bed disability, absence from school, and absence from work. Schools have been sites of major transmission of influenza viruses, and their closure has been considered

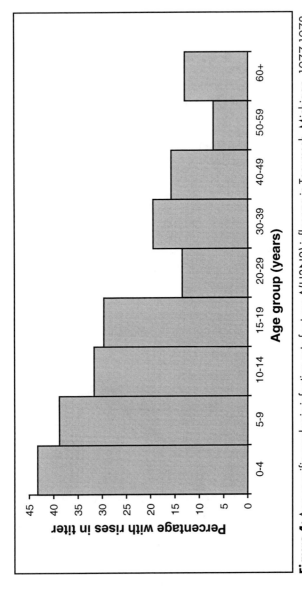

Figure 4: Age-specific serologic infection rate for type A(H3N2) influenza in Tecumseh, Michigan, 1977-1978. There were 835 patients in the study. Monto et al: *Epidemiol Infect* 1993;110:145-160.

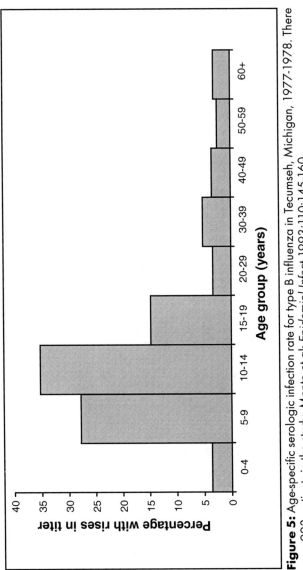

Figure 5: Age-specific serologic infection rate for type B influenza in Tecumseh, Michigan, 1977-1978. There were 993 patients in the study. Monto et al: *Epidemiol Infect* 1993;110:145-160.

69

as a means of stopping outbreaks. However, while school closure should interrupt the outbreak, the need for it is not usually recognized quickly enough for it to have an effect. Also, mechanisms for quick closing of schools are rare; typically, several levels of administrative approval are necessary.

Influenza virus is thought to be transmitted by the airborne aerosol route. This means that it does not need close contact to spread, as the rhinovirus, which produces the common cold, does, and it explains how an influenza virus can pass through a community in 6 to 10 weeks. This is described as a propagated outbreak. Computer simulations of influenza transmission have been carried out as a way to determine the optimal use of vaccine and antivirals. These models become more useful and realistic as more is learned about transmission characteristics; for example, how many people a single person can infect, how many cases of influenza that appear in a household come from other household members, and how many cases of influenza in a household are reintroductions from the community. Reintroductions are possible while the outbreak continues outside the household, and what might appear to be a secondary transmission from parent to child might be a primary transmission from exposure at school. About 40% of infections that appear to be transmitted within a family are brought in from outside.[13] Whether transmission is from within or outside the household is relevant to the use of antiviral drugs in the household.

Other issues that can be studied by transmission modeling include how much each segment of the population contributes to community spread in an influenza outbreak. Because the highest attack rates are in children, it has long been thought that children are responsible for the spread of much of the infection. In some years, illness has peaked first in children, then in adults, and then in nursing home residents. However, in other years, the first indication of increases in influenza transmission has been reporting of an outbreak in a nursing home. Nevertheless, there is no question that children are important in spreading infection. Models have confirmed that it may be possible to reduce the overall community attack rate by vaccinating children. Such an effect was demonstrated during the 1968 A(H3N2) pandemic, when most schoolchildren in one town were administered a new inactivated vaccine before the outbreak began. Transmission in that entire community was reduced by one third.[14] This strategy, confirmed by epidemic modeling, is currently under study with the developmental intranasal live-attenuated vaccine. Reducing transmission is one aim of current vaccination recommendations, but only in limited settings, not for community control. For example, health-care workers and family members of individuals in risk groups should be vaccinated to reduce the likelihood of virus transmission to individuals with underlying disease.

Groups at Risk for Complications

The implications of the term 'risk group' need to be understood in relation to the epidemiology of the disease when discussing control of influenza. Chapter 9 examines this issue in more detail. Children and young adults are at greatest risk of infection. Current influenza vaccination programs are not directed at them as a group, for reasons described elsewhere in this handbook. Rather, influenza vaccination policy concentrates on those who are at high risk of developing complications that might lead to hospitalization and death. Among children this is limited to those 6 months to 2 years of age. These individuals are categorized into risk groups in whom vaccination is clearly cost-effective. These risk groups have been defined by many years of observations and by recent epidemiologic studies. For example, higher mortality in older individuals has been documented in pandemics and epidemics for more than 100 years. The only debate has been whether all persons older than 64 years or only those with defined risk conditions are at higher risk of complications. Two observations led to a universal elderly vaccination policy. One was that many older individuals had undetected underlying conditions that put them at higher risk for complications. The other was evidence that suggested that age functions as a surrogate for other factors leading to risk. Recently, the vaccination recommendation was extended to all persons aged 50 years or older. This was done for programmatic reasons: individuals with underlying risk conditions constitute 30% of this age group, and most were not being vaccinated; vaccination was therefore recommended for the entire group as a way to get the high-risk group vaccinated. Studies on the cost-effectiveness of this strategy are currently under way. Also, recent epidemiologic studies have confirmed observations from pandemics that women, especially in the second and third trimesters of pregnancy, are also at increased risk for influenza complications. Those with underlying cardiovascular disease are at even higher risk. Vaccination is now recommended for all pregnant women.

The Role of Surveillance in Influenza Epidemiology

Surveillance of disease and infection is a major activity. One of its purposes is to detect new viruses of pandemic potential. In interpandemic years, it has many other uses, such as tracking influenza outbreaks: when they start, when they end, and what sort of viral type or subtype is causing them. This information is often of interest to the media and has recently become vital to the appropriate use of antiviral drugs. Surveillance can also estimate the magnitude of an outbreak and characterize its impact. Influenza viruses may spread for several weeks before outbreaks start, and it is necessary to know how many cases are occurring during this period to estimate disease burden. The period during which sporadic viral isolation occurs before an outbreak starts is referred to as 'seeding.' Laboratory and disease surveillance are required to estimate the impact of the subsequent outbreak.

In the United States, laboratory surveillance is provided by a series of World Health Organization (WHO) Influenza Centers, which are typically at hospitals or academic institutions, and by the laboratories of the various state health departments. These laboratories send selected specimens to the influenza branch of the CDC, which also functions as one of four global WHO Influenza Collaborating Centers. This network provides comprehensive information on the kinds of influenza viruses in circulation.[15] The number of isolates being submitted gives a rough indication of the magnitude of the outbreak. These data are supplemented by a growing network of sentinel physicians, who report the number of 'influenza-like illnesses' they see in their practices. Some also collect specimens for virus isolation. Physician-based surveillance of influenza-like illness has been shown to correspond well with data coming from laboratory surveillance.[16] Other countries have different methods for physician-based surveillance. The Royal College of General Practitioners has developed a regular system of medical practice reporting in the United Kingdom that gives a realistic yearly estimate of the impact of influenza and other infectious agents. This system is possible in the United Kingdom because of the organization of medical care there, and it may be possible in other countries with organized health-care systems.

Hospitalization can be a source of surveillance data on influenza occurrence. In the United States, Medicare and Medicaid hospitalization data and data from managed care organizations have been useful in determining the occurrence of severe complications of influenza, but more of the available medical care utilization information should be taken into account. Although information on influenza-related deaths is becoming increasingly accurate, it can be expanded to include additional information on the more severe effects of influenza in general and specific populations.

References

1. Monto AS, Koopman JS, Longini IM Jr: Tecumseh study of illness. XIII. Influenza infection and disease, 1976-1981. *Am J Epidemiol* 1985;121:811-822.

2. Crosby AW. *Epidemic and Peace, 1918.* Westford, CT: Greenwood Press, 1976.

3. Taubenberger JK, Reid AH, Krafft AE, et al: Initial genetic characterization of the 1918 'Spanish' influenza virus. *Science* 1997;275:1793-1796.

4. Monto AS: Influenza: quantifying morbidity and mortality. *Am J Med* 1987;82(suppl 6A):20-25.

5. Martin CJ: An epidemic of fifty cases of influenza among the personnel of a base hospital, B.E.F., France. *Br Med J* 1918:281-282.

6. Simonsen L, Clarke MJ, Schonberger LB, et al: Pandemic versus epidemic influenza mortality: a pattern of changing age distribution. *J Infect Dis* 1998;178:53-60.

7. Chin TD, Foley JF, Doto IL, et al: Morbidity and mortality characteristics of Asian strain influenza. *Public Health Rep* 1960; 75:149-158.

8. Serfling RE: 1963 methods for current statistical analysis of excess pneumonia-influenza deaths. *Public Health Rep* 1963; 78:494-506.

9. Housworth J, Langmuir AD: Excess mortality from epidemic influenza, 1957-1966. *Am J Epidemiol* 1974;100:40-48.

10. Simonsen L, Clarke MJ, Williamson GD, et al: Impact of influenza epidemics on mortality: introducing a severity index. *Am J Public Health* 1997;87:1944-1950.

11. Monto AS, Sullivan KM: Acute respiratory illness in the community. Frequency of illness and the agents involved. *Epidemiol Infect* 1993;110:145-160.

12. Sullivan KM, Monto AS, Longini IM Jr: Estimates of the U.S. health impact of influenza. *Am J Public Health* 1993;83:1712-1716.

13. Monto AS: Interrupting the transmission of respiratory tract infections: theory and practice. *Clin Infect Dis* 1999;28:200-204.

14. Monto AS, Davenport FM, Napier JA, et al: Modification of an outbreak of influenza in Tecumseh, Michigan by vaccination of schoolchildren. *J Infect Dis* 1970;122:16-25.

15. Kendal AP, Joseph JM, Kobayashi G, et al: Laboratory-based surveillance of influenza virus in the United States during the winter of 1977-1978. I. Periods of prevalence of H1N1 and H3N2 influenza strains, their relative rates of isolation in different age groups, and detection of antigenic variants. *Am J Epidemiol* 1979;110: 449-461.

16. Buffington J, Chapman LE, Schmeltz LM, et al: Do family physicians make good sentinels for influenza? *Arch Fam Med* 1993;2:859-864.

6

Chapter 7

Laboratory Diagnosis

A clinical diagnosis of influenza is frequently based on illness characteristics such as abrupt onset, fever, sore throat with dry cough, head and body aches, and reddened, light-sensitive eyes. When properly reported, diagnoses based on illness characteristics can contribute to surveillance programs that track the frequency of influenza-like illness.[1,2]

Laboratory diagnosis of influenza infection has a role in individual patient management, but also serves a public health role. Laboratory diagnosis is particularly useful in special clinical situations, such as in cases with complications and in the immunocompromised. Influenza virus isolation and identification may also be necessary in outbreak investigations and outbreak control. Isolation and antigenic characterization of circulating strains, as part of influenza surveillance programs, are required for epidemiologic investigations and for use in vaccine formulation. Without replicating viruses, it is impossible to produce each year's updated vaccine.

A variety of diagnostic laboratory tests and testing strategies can be used to detect the presence of the virus. In some, viral replication or amplification occurs, and then further methods are used to detect the virus. Other methods directly identify the presence of virus in the collected clinical specimens. Still others use serologic techniques that rely on host immune response to influenza infection with production of antibodies. Rapid diagnostic techniques, such as antigen detection, are appropriate in nursing homes and in primary care or hospital settings where drug intervention opportunities or infection control issues are the focus. Such rapid tests are widely available as kits and require little operator skill or special equipment. These techniques are imperfect, but they contribute a new element to infection recognition.

In contrast, isolation and detailed antigenic characterization of influenza viruses are limited to virus reference laboratories because they require specialized laboratory supplies, equipment, and technical skills. Influenza viruses are typically isolated in mammalian cell cultures or embryonated eggs after inoculation with clinical specimens. Isolation-positive cultures are indicated by the presence of cytopathic effect (CPE), hemagglutination or hemadsorption of red blood cells, and immunostaining techniques. Definitive antigenic characterization requires additional techniques, including hemagglutination inhibition assay (HAI).

Types of Clinical Specimens

Influenza viruses infect respiratory columnar epithelial cells. Throat swabs or nasopharyngeal swabs or washes that sample these infected cells provide suitable specimens for rapid diagnostic tests and cell culture for virus isolation. Specimen collection using cotton or Dacron-tipped swabs should be vigorous, with rotation to obtain cellular material. After collection, swabs should be placed in viral transport medium and agitated to remove cellular material; swabs can then be discarded. Nasal washes are obtained by instilling sterile saline/phosphate buffered saline into nasal passages using a small syringe with fine-bore attached tubing. Saline is immediately suctioned back, and the collected material is placed into vials containing viral transport media. Specimen collection vials are glass or plastic containers, typically with screw caps. Viral transport medium should be a balanced salt solution at neutral pH with protein stabilizers, such as veal infusion broth with bovine serum albumin. Most media include added antibiotics and antifungals to inhibit growth of nonviral respiratory flora.[3] Quality transport media enhance immediate detection of virus and recovery of virus after long-term storage. Specimens should be processed immediately or stored or transported at refrigerator temperatures (4°C) or, for longer periods, frozen to -70°C and shipped in dry ice.

Blood specimens with separation of sera are required for serologic detection of influenza infection; these assays measure or rely on host immune response to infection. Because influenza infection is frequently reinfection with existing partial immunity, current or recent infection status cannot be determined using a single specimen. Instead, paired sera, with the initial specimen collected before or during acute illness and the follow-up specimen collected at least several weeks later, are required for detection of antibody response or change in antibody titer between initial and follow-up specimens. Serologic tests can also be useful in assessing response to vaccination and therefore susceptibility to influenza and as part of epidemiologic surveillance programs.

Primary Viral Isolation in Eggs and Cell Culture

Characterization of the antigenic properties of influenza virus requires amplification of virus in culture systems, including cell monolayers grown on glass or plastic surfaces and in embryonated eggs. These systems permit multiple cycles of viral replication, which result in amplification of virus titer and enhance detection. Several primary and continuous cell lines are susceptible to influenza viruses and permit viral replication, including primary monkey kidney (PMK) and Madin-Darby canine kidney (MDCK).[4,5] Human influenza viruses preferentially attach to cellular sialic acid receptors (with an $\alpha2,6$ linkage to galactose-containing oligosaccharides) present on these and other mammalian cell lines. Replication of influenza viruses requires posttranslational cleavage of the viral hemagglutinin glycoprotein that cannot be accomplished by intracellular proteases during virus assembly in continuous cell lines. As such, the production of infectious progeny virions requires the addition of extraneous proteolytic enzymes, typically trypsin, to cell cultures. PMK cell cultures can support production of infectious virus without addition of trypsin; however, virus growth in these and other culture systems is inhibited by the presence of serum used in cultivation of cell lines. Washing cell cultures with serum-free media before inoculation, plus incubation with serum-free media, maximizes isolation. Primary isolation is also enhanced by use of lower incubation temperatures (33°C), by centrifugation of virus onto cell monolayers, and by rolling tissue culture tubes, where virus-containing culture media washes across cell culture monolayers.

Influenza Isolation in Embryonated Eggs

The traditional way of isolating influenza virus is inoculation of 10- to 11-day-old embryonated hens' eggs. For primary isolation, inoculation into the amniotic sac is required; however, adapted viruses replicate when inoculated allantoically. Typically, the eggs are inoculated blindly; that is, without making a window for direct amniotic inoculation, but simply by inoculating in the direction of the embryo. Egg fluids are harvested after incubation for 3 to 4 days at 33° to 34°C. Egg isolation is still important; all vaccine-candidate viruses must have a history of primary isolation and passage only in eggs. This is done because cell cultures that may be used for isolation are not approved for vaccine production and may contain adventitious agents, which would make the vaccine unacceptable.[6] This is likely going to change, with new cell culture lines being approved for vaccine production.

Identification of Virus Isolation

The presence of influenza viruses in cell culture systems can be detected by a variety of techniques. The CPE typical of both influenza A and B viruses is indicated by the

Table 1: Methods for Detecting Influenza Infection

Viral Propagation and Isolation
- Embryonated eggs
- Cell culture

Direct Antigen Detection in Clinical Specimens
- Polymerase chain reaction
- Rapid antigen detection

Identification of Antibody Response

presence of rounded, refractile, slowly degenerating cells that ultimately detach from the cell monolayer. Detection of CPE is carried out by visually scanning cell monolayers, using a light microscope at low magnification. Unfortunately, CPE may or may not be apparent early in isolation. Therefore, other techniques, including hemadsorption, hemagglutination, and immunostaining, are used to detect virus-infected cells. Hemadsorption and hemagglutination techniques take advantage of the ability of influenza viruses to bind sialic acid residues on the surface of red blood cells of various species, including guinea pigs and chickens. With hemadsorption, red blood cells attach to the surface of infected monolayers in the presence of viral hemagglutinin glycoproteins on the cell membranes of infected cells.[7] Red cell attachment is visualized microscopically for easy identification of positive cultures; agglutinated red blood cells may also be seen floating in culture media.

Hemadsorption inhibition can also be used to type isolates. Addition of specific antisera can be used to prevent the adherence of the red cells. This technique is rarely used because of the availability of other methods (Table 1). In the presence of influenza virus in suspension, red blood cells agglutinate (hemagglutination), forming a lattice that falls to the bottom of a tube or plate in a characteristic pattern. These techniques are widely used in diagnostic laboratories to screen cell systems inoculated with clinical specimens for influenza (and other viruses). The same method is used subsequently as part of virus typing. A major disadvantage of these techniques to detect virus presence is the time required to determine culture-positive status, typically 4 to 5 days. Associated costs and time can be reduced and the manipulation of large numbers of clinical specimens can be made easier with the use of shell vials or multiwell (96-well) plates. With these systems, MDCK cells are seeded on shell vial slides or multiwell plates; when monolayers are confluent (monolayer covering entire surface), clinical specimens are inoculated with centrifugation of the clinical material onto the cell culture for improved sensitivity. Cultures are incubated at 33° to 35°C for 12 to 72 hours and then processed using immunostaining techniques for evidence of influenza-specific proteins. Complete antigenic characterization is not possible with these cost- and time-efficient methods and requires traditional isolation in macrosystems.

Type-Specific Identification of Influenza

Once virus presence is identified, the next step is to confirm that the virus is influenza and to type it (Table 2). Immunostaining techniques, including immunofluorescent assays (IFAs) or enzyme immunoassays (EIAs), can be directly applied to respiratory specimens containing exfoliated cells and to cell culture systems (culture tubes, shell vials, or multiwell plates) either before (earlier in the isolation process) or after visualization of CPE or testing for hemadsorption or hemagglutination. These techniques can differentiate between influenza types A and B as well as influenza isolates from other viruses (parainfluenza viruses). These other viruses may circulate at the same time,

> **Table 2: Methods Used to Identify Viral Type or Subtype**
>
> *Virus Identification*
> - Immunofluorescence (IFM)
> - Enzyme immunoassay (EIA)
> - Hemagglutination inhibition assay (HI or HAI)
> - Hemadsorption inhibition
> - Neutralization
>
> *Serology*
> - Hemagglutination inhibition assay (HI or HAI)
> - Neutralization
> - Enzyme-linked immunosorbent assay (ELISA)

grow preferentially in PMK cells, and be characterized by hemadsorption. Using IFA techniques, exfoliated cells from respiratory specimens or cells scraped from monolayers are applied to microscope slides and fixed using acetone; shell vials and monolayers in multiwell plates need only be fixed. Cell preparations are reacted with commercially available specific antibodies, typically monoclonal antibodies (commonly produced in mice) to conserved areas of influenza proteins (NP or M1 proteins). These monoclonal antibodies are either directly conjugated to a fluorochrome or reacted with a second antispecies (goat antimouse) antibody conjugated to a fluorochrome.[8,9] In the presence of influenza-infected cells, fluorochrome-labeled areas are observed using a fluorescence microscope. Enzyme immunoassay techniques use the same principle of antibody-conjugated label, but in this case the label is an enzyme indicator molecule. The reaction of this enzyme label, when specifically attached to influenza-infected cells in culture, with substrate yields a colorimetric reaction that is observed visually or detected with an automated reader.[10]

The IFA and EIA techniques will separate viruses into type A or B. However, they will not distinguish between type A(H3N2) and type A(H1N1). Differentiation between influenza A subtypes and identification of antigenic drift of type A and B viruses are traditionally done using HAI techniques. This technique takes advantage of the influenza phenomenon of hemagglutination, which can be inhibited to a degree determined by the antigenic similarity between the influenza test strain and the various strains used to develop specific neutralizing antisera. In this assay, specific antisera, produced in ferrets, sheep, or chickens, are titrated using doubling dilutions and incubated with influenza viruses of unknown antigenic type.[11] Inhibition at the highest tested dilution would indicate antigenic identity; no inhibition would indicate separate influenza types (A vs B) and subtypes (H1N1 vs H3N2). Greater or lesser inhibition suggests novel circulating varieties or antigenic drift within influenza subtypes. The related hemadsorption inhibition technique may also be used to subtype viruses (see above). This is now rarely used, as is the neutralization technique.

Detection of Viral RNA

Reverse transcriptase (RT)-polymerase chain reaction (PCR) techniques have recently been applied to diagnosis, typing, and subtyping of influenza virus in clinical material or tissue culture fluids. Because of their sensitivity, these techniques can be applied to viral detection in clinical specimens without amplification in cell culture. In this procedure, viral RNA is extracted and reverse transcribed.[12] Complementary DNA is amplified in the presence of multiple selected primers capable of differentiating between influenza types and subtypes, followed by agarose gel electrophoresis and ethidium bromide staining. Visible electrophoretic patterns are compared to those of control specimens to determine antigenic identity. The 'nested' PCR procedure adds a second amplification step with a second set of primers that sit down inside the sequence created by the first amplification; this additional step increases the procedure's sensitivity. With appropriate primer selection, this molecular technique can be applied to circulating influenza strains to improve the quality of surveillance data for annual vaccine formulation and outbreak investigations and can be applied to differentiation of reassortant vaccine strains from wild-type strains for use in newer vaccine development. DNA sequencing of PCR products can provide information on variation of influenza viruses, including sequence changes associated with antigenic drift and those associated with antiviral resistance. RT-PCR tests can be costly and require advanced technical skill to perform. Newer PCR procedures are more rapid (called real-time PCR) and are less likely to have technical problems but require special equipment. These procedures are likely to become standard in specialized laboratories, and, for example, are currently in use to rapidly identify H5 avian viruses.

Rapid Detection Techniques

The development of rapid techniques is relatively new for influenza detection. The techniques already described require days for viral detection (isolation) or are complicated and expensive laboratory methods (PCR). The rapid techniques use a variety of methods that have been simplified so that they can be applied in most laboratories or, in some cases, at the bedside. These new techniques involve miniaturization and increased sensitivity. Amplification takes place ordinarily in eggs or cell culture or within the PCR technique. It is no surprise, therefore, that the major debate about the appropriate use of rapid techniques involves their sensitivity. Basically, the more virus that is shed, the more sensitive the technique. Therefore, these techniques have been most useful in young children. That is why the method for respiratory syncytial virus detection has been so successful.

Several basic methods have been used in designing the rapid tests. The EIA technique has most frequently been modified as an enzyme immunomembrane filter assay. In the Directigen™ influenza test, clinical specimens are diluted with buffer containing a mucolytic agent and applied to a filter membrane. Viral antigens, if present, are nonspecifically absorbed to the membrane, followed by specific detection (influenza A or B) using monoclonal antibodies linked to chromogens. Positive results are indicated by the presence of the visible pattern (triangle shape) as a result of the colorimetric reaction.[13]

Other techniques use modifications of the EIA method but different ways to indicate that a positive reaction has taken place. In the flu optical immunoassay (FLU OIA) method, a mirror-like surface of a silicon wafer is coated with an optical thin film and captures antibody specific for type A and B influenza. Antigen-antibody complexing is detected through horseradish peroxidase-congregated antibody. Positivity is indicated in the wafer by development of a purple spot. Type A and B positivity are not distinguished. The test takes approximately 20 minutes to perform.[14]

The QuickVue® similarly depends on antibody-antigen reaction and does not distinguish between type A and B. It is waived under the Clinical Laboratory Improvement Act (CLIA), which means that it can be performed at the bedside.

Somewhat different is the Zstat™ test. This method is based on the detection of the neuraminidase activity of the influenza virus. Unlike the QuickVue® test, the Zstat™ test can be performed on throat swabs. It is also CLIA waived.

Thus, different types of specimens and different types of swabs are required for each of these tests. The instructions should be followed for optimal performance. Manufacturers also provide information on the sensitivity and specificity of their tests.[15] It must be assumed that these results were achieved using optimal specimens and may not be replicated in actual conditions.

In determining how to use these tests appropriately, their cost, sensitivity, and specificity must be considered. These are examined in Chapter 16. Reports of sensitivity have varied greatly in comparative studies. In a study conducted by a state health department laboratory using one test, sensitivity was found to be 40%.[16] This possible lower sensitivity should be factored into the way the tests are used and is not particularly troublesome. Of greater concern are reports, some anecdotal, of the tests' lack of specificity. This has been rare under highly controlled conditions but appears to be more common under circumstances of actual use. Sensitivity and specificity issues indicate that it is not appropriate to use these tests to make a diagnosis of influenza in an individual patient. Rather, the tests should be used selectively to confirm, for example, that influenza is in a geographic area or institution. In any event, other laboratory techniques should still be used for clear confirmation.

Serologic Diagnosis of Influenza

Serologic diagnosis of influenza does not have a role in the immediate clinical management of illnesses because of the need for paired sera. Serologic studies do contribute to influenza surveillance programs by providing retrospective determination of influenza activity and by determining immunologic response to vaccination. Hemagglutination inhibition is the most frequently used serologic test for influenza infection. Sera are pretreated with heat and receptor-destroying enzyme to reduce nonspecific inhibition. In multiwell plates, sera samples are serially diluted with doubling dilutions and incubated with standard doses of virus antigens. After incubation, guinea pig or chick red blood cells are added and allowed to sediment. Plates are tipped, and red blood cells that have settled will produce a streak (red blood cells run/flow), indicating inhibition of hemagglutination and antigenic identity between the strain responsible for immune response and a known influenza test strain. Wells with lattice formation (hemagglutination) will not streak. When processing paired sera, an antibody response, or change in antibody titers between initial and follow-up specimens, indicates exposure to that specific strain as a result of infection or response to vaccination. An HAI antibody titer of ≥40 postvaccination is generally taken as an indication of protection from subsequent infection.[17]

Neutralization assays using enzyme immunoassays are also suitable for titration of neutralizing antibodies or detection of antibody titer change between paired sera. With this technique, sera at varying dilutions are mixed with virus strains of interest and transferred onto monolayers of MDCK cells in multiwell plates. After an incubation period for virus replication, cells are fixed and stained for influenza-infected cells using specific monoclonal antibodies conjugated to enzyme. The addition of substrate yields a colorimetric reaction that can be evaluated using spectrophotometric absorbance to determine change in neutralizing activity between paired sera or activity above cut points. Other methods have been used for detecting whether neutralization has taken place. The neutralization test has been particularly important in detecting antibodies to the avian viruses in the 1997 Hong Kong outbreak. Antibody detection in these situations with HAI has not been good. This may also prove to be a problem in evaluating vaccines to avian antigens. The EIA technique may also be used directly for antibody detection using, for example, purified hemagglutinin attached to a surface. The method would then be similar to that used for detecting an unknown antigen.

Summary

Rapid diagnostic tests may play an increasingly important role in influenza diagnosis because of the availability of effective influenza antiviral drugs used as either treatment or prophylaxis. Management of illness in individual patients and control of institutional outbreaks (nursing homes) will benefit from rapid diagnostic techniques. However, these techniques need to be to used with caution and, for now, should be used more to confirm the presence of influenza in a community rather than in each patient seen. However, isolation and antigenic characterization of circulating strains using a variety of techniques will still be required for annual epidemiologic surveillance and for use in vaccine formulation.

References

1.   Monto AS, Gravenstein S, Elliott M, et al: Clinical signs and symptoms predicting influenza infection. *Arch Intern Med* 2000; 160:3243-3247.

2.   Boivin G, Hardy I, Tellier G, et al: Predicting influenza infections during epidemics with use of a clinical case definition. *Clin Infect Dis* 2000;31:1166-1169.

3.   Monto AS, Ohmit SE, Margulies JR, et al: Medical practice-based influenza surveillance: viral prevalence and assessment of morbidity. *Am J Epidemiol* 1995;141:502-506.

4.   Tobita K, Sugiura A, Enomote C, et al: Plaque assay and primary isolation of influenza A viruses in an established line of canine kidney cells (MDCK) in the presence of trypsin. *Med Microbiol Immunol* 1975;162:9-14.

5.   Govorkova EA, Murti G, Meignier B, et al: African green monkey kidney (Vero) cells provide an alternative host system for influenza A and B viruses. *J Virol* 1996;70:5519-5524.

6.   Monto AS, Maassab HF, Bryan ER: Relative efficacy of embryonated eggs and cell culture for isolation of contemporary influenza viruses. *J Clin Microbiol* 1981;13:233-235.

7.   Shelokov A, Vogel JE, Chi L: Hemadsorption (adsorption-hemagglutination) test for viral agents in tissue culture with special reference to influenza. *Proc Soc Exp Biol Med* 1958;97:802-809.

8.   Johansson ME, Grandien M, Arro L: Preparation of sera for subtyping of influenza A viruses by immunofluorescence. *J Immunol Methods* 1979;27:263-272.

9.   Sarkkinen HK, Halonen PE, Salmi AA: Detection of influenza A virus by radioimmunoassay and enzyme-immunoassay from nasopharyngeal specimens. *J Med Virol* 1981;7:213-220.

10. Julkunen I, Pyhala R, Hovi T: Enzyme immunoassay, complement fixation and hemagglutination inhibition tests in the diagnosis of influenza A and B virus infections. Purified hemagglutinin in subtype-specific diagnosis. *J Virol Methods* 1985;10:75-84.

11. Hirst GK: The quantitative determination of influenza virus and antibodies by means of red cell agglutination. *J Exp Med* 1942; 74:47-64.

12. Ellis JS, Fleming DM, Zambon MC: Multiplex reverse transcription-PCR for surveillance of influenza A and B viruses in England and Wales in 1995 and 1996. *J Clin Microbiol* 1997;35: 2076-2082.

13. Waner JL, Todd SJ, Shalaby H, et al: Comparison of Directigen FLU-A with viral isolation and direct immunofluorescence for the rapid detection and identification of influenza A virus. *J Clin Microbiol* 1991;29:479-482.

14. Herrmann B, Larsson C, Zweygberg BW: Simultaneous detection and typing of influenza viruses A and B by a nested reverse transcription-PCR: comparison to virus isolation and antigen detection by immunofluorescence and optical immunoassay (FLU OIA). *J Clin Microbiol* 2001;39:134-138.

15. Rapid diagnostic tests for influenza. *Med Lett Drugs Ther* 1999; 41:121-122.

16. Effler PV, Ieong MC, Tom T, et al: Enhancing public health surveillance for influenza virus by incorporating newly available rapid diagnostic tests. *Emerg Infect Dis* 2002;8:23-28.

17. Hobson D, Curry RL, Beare AS, et al: The role of serum haemagglutination-inhibiting antibody in protection against challenge infection with influenza A2 and B viruses. *J Hyg (Lond)* 1972;70: 767-777.

Chapter **8**

Ecology of Influenza

Influenza infects many different mammalian and avian species but only causes disease in some. This wide-spread dissemination in nature is limited to type A viruses; type B viruses are restricted to humans but have recently been reported in seals, probably as a result of human-to-seal transmission and further spread from seal to seal. The ecology of type A influenza, as shown in Figure 1, is important for two reasons. First, influenza can create economic loss when it infects horses, chickens, and turkeys. Second, and more importantly, influenza in animals transmits to humans and almost certainly can produce a pandemic after reassorting with a human virus.[1]

Equine Influenza

Equine influenza, which has little confirmed relation to human influenza, has a major economic impact, especially when racehorses are infected. It is the animal influenza viral infection that bears the closest clinical resemblance to human influenza. It is a respiratory illness with denudation of the ciliated epithelium and, often, bronchitis, bronchiolitis, and interstitial pneumonia. The horses experience fever, dyspnea, and cough and may be incapacitated for weeks.[2] The disease has been recognized for centuries, but the viruses themselves, A(H7N7) and A(H3N8), were first isolated from horses in 1956. Some inconclusive evidence that the influenza in humans at the end of the 19th century was caused by an H3N8 virus has resulted in a hypothesis that the equine virus was transferred to humans. Contradict-

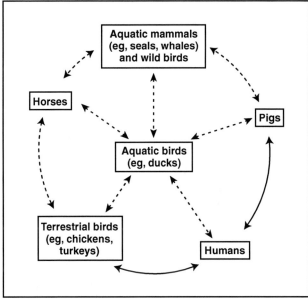

Figure 1: The 'wheel of flu.' The working hypothesis is that wild aquatic birds are the primordial reservoir of all type A influenza viruses of avian and mammalian species. Transmission of influenza has been demonstrated between pigs and humans and now between chickens and humans (solid line). There is excellent circumstantial evidence for transmission of influenza between aquatic birds and some of the other species shown (dotted lines). Evidence for transmission between other species has not yet been established. Adapted from Ito T, Kawaoka Y: Avian influenza. In: Nicholson KG, Webster R, Hay A, eds. *Textbook of Influenza*. Oxford: Blackwell Science, 1998.

ing evidence suggests that both viruses originated from an avian source at the same time.

Because of its economic importance, equine influenza has been the subject of surveillance for many years, but often in more isolation than the surveillance of animal viruses thought to be more closely related to human influenza. The epizootiology has been followed carefully. As with some avian viruses, the equine A(H3N8) viruses have split into American and Eurasian lineages. Inactivated vaccine for the equine lineages was introduced in the late 1960s, and different formulations and vaccination schedules are now in use. Horses are moved from country to country for racing events, and international regulations require the animals to be vaccinated to prevent the spread of the virus. Various vaccine strategies, including the use of 'naked' DNA, have been explored experimentally. The M2 inhibitors have been used successfully in treatment to reduce symptoms, but with little effect on virus shedding.[3]

Swine Influenza

The first influenza virus to be isolated from any species was recovered from pigs in 1930. The virus causes clinical symptoms in infected animals; however, at least in the United States, it is not severe enough and does not have enough economic importance to necessitate the development of a vaccine. Swine influenza is a respiratory syndrome with labored breathing, fever, nasal discharge, and conjunctivitis. There is some weight loss, but the disease lasts only 5 to 7 days, with complete recovery. This syndrome led to the recognition of the disease in the American Midwest in 1918. Based on the timing of this observation and the occurrence of the human pandemic in the same year, it has been assumed that the human virus entered the swine population at that time. This A(H1N1) virus, termed classical swine influenza, was isolated from a pig in Iowa in 1930 and has infected pigs, in some form, ever since.[4]

The North American A(H1N1) virus was introduced into Asia in the 1970s. American swine viruses have also been introduced into Europe but have been largely replaced by A(H1N1) viruses of avian origin, suggesting that avian viruses can more easily transmit directly into pigs than into humans. Another example of the ease of direct transmission of viruses into pigs was the appearance of the A(H3N2) virus in pigs in East Asia and Hawaii shortly after it started to transmit in humans in the late 1960s. These viruses did not produce a clinical disease in infected pigs and did not become established in swine in the United States.[5]

A study of the evolution of the swine viruses over time demonstrates that, similar to the findings with equine and human viruses, in the face of antibody pressure, the viruses change continually. The rate of such changes has been followed, the evolution of the viruses has been charted with phylogenetic trees, and clusters of viruses of similar structure have been identified. In contrast, changes in avian viruses in birds have been slow. Because pigs can be infected by viruses from many species, they have been referred to as 'mixing vessels,' in which coinfection by viruses from various species can theoretically produce new viruses through reassortment.[6]

Avian Influenza

As shown in Table 1, a limited number of hemagglutinins are found in human, swine, and equine influenza viruses. The same is true of the various neuraminidases, of which only two, N1 and N2, have been found in humans, although N8 may have been present in the past. In contrast, all 16 hemagglutinins and 9 neuraminidases exist among various domestic and wild birds. Some infect with no symptoms; in other situations, lethal disease occurs.[7] The infection can be widespread with the involvement of multiple organs or can be much more limited. However, what is common to many species is that the viruses infect the cells of the gastrointestinal tract and are shed into the feces and, for aquatic birds, into the water, from which they can be recovered.[8] Viruses shed over months from healthy aquatic birds can infect other species, particularly chickens. Chickens and turkeys, in contrast to aquatic birds, may develop potentially severe disease when infected. Some

Table 1: Distribution of Influenza Hemagglutinins in Nature

	Birds	Humans	Swine	Horses
H1	+	+	+	-
H2	+	+	-	-
H3	+	+	+	+
H4	+	-	-	-
H5	+	?	-	-
H6	+	-	-	-
H7	+	-	-	+
H8	+	-	-	-
H9	+	?	-	-
H10-16	+	-	-	-

particular strains are more virulent for one species than the other, but both species can experience major outbreaks with viruses of certain hemagglutinins and neuraminidases, with considerable economic impact.

Viruses that contain H5 and H7 have been the ones most involved with virulent outbreaks of disease in poultry. The classic virus of fowl plague, an H7N1 virus, is highly virulent in chickens and turkeys, with an extremely low dose of virus required to produce infection. High virulence in poultry appears to be associated with the cleavability of the viral hemagglutinin,[9] which is necessary for viral replication. The exact amino acids involved in rendering the hemagglutinin cleavable have been mapped, and this has been useful in evaluating the recent outbreaks of A(H5N1), a virus that contained a multibasic cleavage site.

The transmission of the virulent viruses in poultry seems to vary in terms of the specific virus involved. These viruses sometimes do not spread as widely as avirulent ones because of their rapid lethality, which kills the birds that could further disseminate the virus. In the past, outbreaks of the lethal viruses were often self-limited and self-extinguishing and, sometimes, were helped along by massive slaughter of the exposed birds; this has a major economic impact. In 1983-1984, before a virulent H5N2 outbreak could be controlled, more than 17 million birds had to be destroyed. Recent outbreaks of highly pathogenic H5- and H7-containing viruses have had a major social and economic impact. As a result, vaccines for poultry have been developed. The M2-inhibiting antivirals have also been used in these outbreaks, but they have had limited success because of the development of resistant viruses.

Relationship of Avian Viruses to Human Disease

Strong evidence suggests that human type A viruses originally came from birds. The antigenic stability of the viruses in birds and their wide distribution suggest that, at some time in the remote past, the viruses moved into mammals, in whom they are less stable. More recent human pandemic viruses also probably had their origin in birds. Such viruses can be produced by mutation or by reassortment, in which an avian virus and a human virus coinfect a host and exchange gene segments to produce a new virus. This is possible because the viral genome is segmented. All that is necessary for a virus of pandemic potential to emerge is for the human virus to acquire the hemagglutinin, or the hemagglutinin and neuraminidase, from the avian strain; however, other segments may be acquired as well.

One major problem with this hypothetic scenario is that avian viruses were thought to be unable to infect humans directly (which is one reason why the events of 1997 in Hong Kong and elsewhere in susequent years came as such a surprise), and human strains were thought to be unable to infect birds directly. The molecular explanation for this inability to infect other species is differences in the receptor specificity of the hemagglutinin of avian and human virus. Avian virus hemagglutinins bind preferentially with the sialic acid-α2,3-galactose linkage, while human virus hemagglutinins bind with the α2,6-galactose linkage. Epithelial cells in duck intestines, where the avian viruses bind, contain α2,3-galactose linkage, not the α2,6 that is present in human respiratory epithelium. However, the epithelial cells of swine contain both linkages, making pigs mixing vessels where reassortment of avian and human viruses can take place.[10]

Interspecies Transmission of Avian Viruses

Because ducks and related aquatic birds shed virus of different hemagglutinins and neuraminidases for long periods, and because they are in contact with various terrestrial birds, such as chickens and turkeys, and with various mammals, they have been thought to be the natural reservoir of influenza viruses. Because transmission in animals is impossible to observe, it is usually assumed to have taken place when a virus with specific antigenic characteristics is found first in one species and later in another. Sometimes, the first virus is isolated in one geographic area and the later one is isolated in another area, so there is uncertainty about the event itself. Much of the doubt has been removed in recent years by new molecular techniques in which amino acids can be sequenced and viruses can be identified as having an avian or mammalian lineage. These techniques have also made it possible to divide avian lineages into American and Eurasian. Using these molecular methods, it is now possible to say that the 1957 pandemic virus A(H2N2), arising in China, received three gene segments, a polymerase and the hemagglutinin and neuraminidase coding genes, from a Eurasian avian virus. In 1968, a similar event occurred, but only the first two genes came from a Eurasian avian virus. In this case, the new virus, A(H3N2), retained the neuraminidase of the previously circulating human virus. It is hypothesized that this reassortment took place in pigs.[11,12] More recently, it has been demonstrated that the 1918 virus derived from an unknown avian ancestor, not by reassortment but by mutation.

Surveillance of the Ecology of Influenza Viruses

Because of the evidence that avian influenza viruses can spread to humans after reassortment in pigs, increased attention has been paid to the study of this interaction in recent years. Particular attention has been paid to East Asia, where the new pandemic viruses have emerged and where aquatic birds, pigs, and humans live in close proximity to each other, which would make transmission and reassortment more likely. Given the vast number of birds and large numbers of pigs, the study of influenza in these species is a useful exercise but is sometimes of questionable relevance to human disease. However, the occurrence of influenza in the human populations in contact with these animals is critical. While it is most likely that new viruses of epidemiologic importance will arise in East Asia, it is not certain, so efforts to follow the human-animal interaction in terms of transmission need to be expanded to other regions. These types of studies are important so that they can give an early warning concerning the emergence of a new pandemic virus. Only contrasting studies of human populations and animal populations will identify viruses that have the potential for cross-species transmission. Simply identifying a virus in a bird or a mammal does not reveal anything about the capacity of the virus to spread to humans.

In 1999, workers in China and Hong Kong identified an A(H9N2) virus of avian origin infecting humans.[13] This identification provided a 'wake-up call' to initiate more extensive surveillance to determine if further transmission was taking place. Such transmission was not documented, but this virus is still one of particular interest for pandemic preparation.

An example of viral spread that is of interest, but not major consequence, to public health involves the transmission of viruses to mammals such as seals and whales.[14] These mammals are in close contact with aquatic birds, and transmission of avian viruses might be facilitated by exposure to the birds' droppings. Repeated isolation of type A influenza in seals and whales has been reported; however, the infection does not seem to be of particular consequence to humans. In other words, unlike pigs, these mammals do not appear to have a role as a mixing vessel for human infection.

Avian Influenza in Asia, beginning in 1997

In 1997, a momentous event took place in Hong Kong that, in many ways, revolutionized the role of avian influenza infection in human disease. In May, a single case of influenza was reported in a child, and, eventually, this illness was found to be an infection with the avian H5N1 influenza.[13] This virus was recognized as one that caused severe, lethal disease in poultry but, according to the existing belief, could not spread to humans. The fact that the child in question was immunocompromised was considered by some to explain the transmission. However, months later, cases in humans started to occur in conjunction with the return of the A(H5N1) infection in chickens in the live-bird markets of Hong Kong. The second wave of human infection involved individuals with no heightened susceptibility. One aspect of this outbreak was consistent with a long-term belief: the virus that invaded the chickens seemed to come from geese, the aquatic-bird reservoir.

An initial solution in Hong Kong was to separate the live-bird markets handling terrestrial birds from those handling aquatic birds. The direct infection of humans with an unchanged avian virus was unexpected and did not follow the theories of the receptor specificity of each of those strains. However, the avian viruses did not appear capable of further human-to-human transmission. With the return of these viruses to many countries in 2003, human-to-human transmission continues to be limited, and the viruses fully retain avian characteristics. These events are described in greater detail in Chapter 15.

References

1. Kilbourne E: Recombination of influenza A viruses of human and animal origin. *Science* 1968;160:74-76.

2. Gerber H: Clinical features, sequelae, and epidemiology of equine influenza. In: Bryans JT, Gerber H, eds. *Equine Infectious Diseases II.* Basel, S. Karger, pp 63-80, 1970.

3. Rees WA, Harkins JD, Woods WE, et al: Amantadine and equine influenza: pharmacology, pharmacokinetics and neurological effects in the horse. *Equine Vet J* 1997;29:104-110.

4. Shope RD: Swine influenza. III. Filtration experiments and aetiology. *J Exp Med* 1931;54:373-385.

5. Schultz U, Fitch WM, Ludwig S, et al: Evolution of pig influenza viruses. *Virology* 1991;183:61-73.

6. Scholtissek C. Pigs as 'mixing vessels' for the creation of new pandemic influenza A viruses. *Med Principles Pract* 1990;2:65-71.

7. Kawaoka Y, Nestorowicz A, Alexander DJ, et al: Molecular analyses of the hemagglutinin genes of H5 influenza viruses: origin of a virulent turkey strain. *Virology* 1987;158:218-227.

8. Webster RG, Yakhno M, Hinshaw VS, et al: Intestinal influenza: replication and characterization of influenza viruses in ducks. *Virology* 1978;84:268-278.

9. Li SQ, Orlich M, Rott R: Generation of seal influenza virus variants pathogenic for chickens, because of hemagglutinin cleavage site changes. *J Virol* 1990;64:3297-3303.

10. Rogers GN, Paulson JC: Receptor determinants of human and animal influenza virus isolates: differences in receptor specificity of the H3 hemagglutinin based on species of origin. *Virology* 1983;127:361-373.

11. Scholtissek C, Rohde W, Von Hoyningen V, et al: On the origin of the human influenza virus subtypes H2N2 and H3N2. *Virology* 1978;87:13-20.

12. Kawaoka Y, Krauss S, Webster RG: Avian-to-human transmission of the PB1 gene of influenza A viruses in the 1957 and 1968 pandemics. *J Virol* 1989;63:4603-4608.

13. Guan Y, Shortridge KF, Krauss S, et al: Molecular characterization of H9N2 influenza viruses: were they the donors of the 'internal' genes of H5N1 viruses in Hong Kong? *Proc Natl Acad Sci U S A* 1999; 96:9363-9367.

14. Webster RG, Hinshaw VS, Bean WJ, et al: Characterization of an influenza A virus from seals. *Virology* 1981;113:712-724.

Chapter 9

Inactivated Vaccine and Its Use

The current inactivated influenza vaccine was developed during World War II. The work was carried out under the auspices of the US Armed Forces. With the high morbidity associated with an influenza outbreak, there was concern that troops could be rendered unfit for service, with disastrous consequences.[1] The Armed Forces Commission on Influenza continued to take the lead in evaluating vaccines until approximately 1969, when the overall direction was assumed by the National Institutes of Health. Throughout this period, the vaccine was evaluated on an almost annual basis in large-scale, placebo-controlled trials. Results of many of these trials are shown in Figure 1. Each year, the vaccine was found to be 70% to 90% effective in preventing laboratory-confirmed clinical influenza.[2] An exception was in 1955, when the virus in the vaccine did not match (ie, did not resemble closely enough) the virus causing the outbreak. The result was much lower clinical efficacy.

The lessons learned from the military trials can be carried forward to the present. The vaccines produced from 1943 to 1969 are similar to those now in use, at least in terms of basic production and inactivation. Therefore, the efficacy of 70% to 90% is still the one quoted for today's vaccines. The need for a close similarity in surface antigens, particularly the hemagglutinin, between the virus in the vaccine and the one circulating continues.

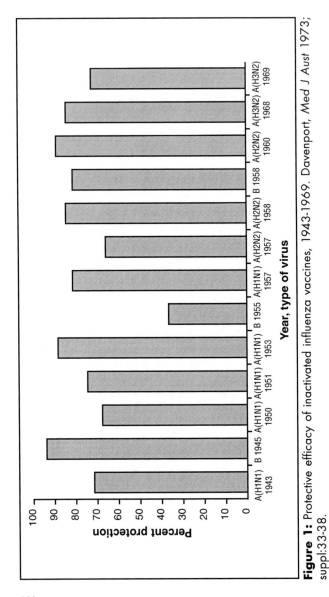

Figure 1: Protective efficacy of inactivated influenza vaccines, 1943-1969. Davenport, *Med J Aust* 1973; suppl:33-38.

The early vaccines, similar to the present ones, were prepared by inoculating fertile hens' eggs amniotically. The product was then formalinized to inactivate the virus; that is, to render it noninfectious. To produce the vaccine, methods were developed to concentrate the virus so that there would be sufficient antigenic mass in the inoculum to produce an antibody response. However, the process also concentrated egg proteins and other viral components not needed to produce immunity to the hemagglutinin and the neuraminidase. The reactogenicity produced by these vaccines was a problem, especially in young children. Current vaccines do not cause the same level of reactogenicity. Zonal centrifugation allowed purification of the virus particles, further removing the egg proteins;[3] the result was what is now termed a *whole virus vaccine*.

In the late 1950s, ether treatment was discovered to disrupt the influenza virus, resulting in a preparation that was still immunogenic but less reactogenic.[4] Other splitting agents have been developed and, combined with processes such as rate zonal centrifugation, produce a highly pure preparation of hemagglutinin and neuraminidase. It was shown in the 1976 swine influenza trials that children required split vaccines to avoid reactogenicity.[5] However, the whole virus had a priming effect, and two doses of the split vaccine had to be given in unprimed children. For many years, the vaccines used in the United States have been almost exclusively split.

The current vaccines also have a higher antigenic content than some of the older ones, in which standardization was inconsistent. The first major advance was the use of hemagglutination to determine concentration of the hemagglutinin antigen. However, it was demonstrated that this technique could vary twofold from laboratory to laboratory. Unreliability was increased depending on whether whole virus or split vaccine was assayed. Therefore, techniques such as single radial immunodiffusion and rocket immunoelectrophoresis were introduced. These techniques, or variants thereof, are now in use to standardize the amount of hemagglutinin in the vaccine at 15 mg per antigen.[6] Neuraminidase is not standardized.

Selection of Viruses for the Vaccine

The influenza vaccine contains representatives of all influenza viruses circulating somewhere in the world. This means that each year, two A viruses, A(H3N2) and A(H1N1), must be included in the vaccine, as well as a type B virus. Because the hemagglutinin and, to a lesser extent, the neuraminidase in each virus change from year to year (a process known as antigenic drift), the viruses in the vaccine must be reviewed every year to determine their closeness to those causing outbreaks somewhere in the world. When there is a divergence, a new virus must be chosen. This happens most often for A(H3N2), which changes more rapidly than the other virus types or subtypes. The decision for the northern hemisphere is made at a meeting held each year in February at the World Health Organization (WHO), and a US meeting held by the Food and Drug Administration (FDA). A second WHO meeting is held each year in October for the southern hemisphere. The two WHO meetings emphasize the need for the most up-to-date information. Information considered at these meetings includes immunologic comparisons of relationships among strains causing outbreaks around the world and new data from the sequencing of the hemagglutinin. Surveillance and representation of all influenza viruses are therefore important.

The decision of which viruses to include in the vaccine is usually relatively straightforward. However, in some years, there may be two different varieties of a subtype circulating. The hope is to choose a virus that produces immunity against both, but this is not always possible. There is also an effort to choose a strain that will grow well in eggs. Some flexibility is usually included with that point in mind. Thus, the recommendations generally specify that the virus be, for example, 'A/California/07/2004(H3N2)-like,' the 'like' introducing the element of flexibility.

Vaccine for North America is produced from February to the subsequent autumn. Because all three strains have to be produced separately and then combined, manufacturers often start earlier, after checking informally with, in the United States, the US Food and Drug Administration or the Centers for Disease Control and Prevention (CDC) to determine which of the previous year's viruses will probably remain the same. Rarely, there is a change in the circulating virus late in the process or even after the vaccine is released. The last time a significant change took place was in 2003-2004, when the A/Fujian/411/2002(H3N2) strains emerged, and were only partially inhibited by the vaccine, which protected against A/Panama/2007/99(H3N2).

ACIP Recommendations for Use of Influenza Vaccine

Policy for use of vaccine in the United States is set by the Advisory Committee on Immunization Practices (ACIP); for certain specific vaccines, professional groups such as the American Academy of Pediatrics also issue recommendations (the Red Book). Policy on use of influenza vaccine has evolved gradually over time. Among the most recent additions to the risk groups recommended to receive vaccine are women who will be pregnant during the influenza season. Vaccination can occur during any trimester. The importance of influenza in young children has also been recognized recently. Recommendations are based on evidence of added health risk in a particular group and, if data are available, on evidence that prevention of illness is cost-effective. In the past, when inactivated vaccine was the only preparation available in the United States, all US recommendations referred to that vaccine. Now that a live-attenuated vaccine is available, the ACIP has issued specific recommendations for its use. Chapter

Table 1: Target Groups of Persons to Be Vaccinated for Their Own Protection

- Adults older than 49 years (previously older than 64 years)
- Residents of nursing homes and residents with chronic conditions in other facilities
- Adults and children with chronic disorders of the pulmonary or cardiovascular system, including asthma
- Adults and children with chronic metabolic diseases (including diabetes mellitus), renal dysfunction, hemoglobinopathies, or immuno-suppression (including those immunosuppressed by medication)
- Children and teenagers (6 months to 18 years) who are on long-term aspirin therapy
- Women who will be pregnant during the influenza season
- People with any condition that compromises res-piratory function or the handling of respiratory secretions, or that can increase the risk for aspira-tion (eg, people with cognitive dysfunction, spinal cord injuries, seizure disorders, or other neuro-muscular disorders)
- Children age 6 to 23 months

10 provides information on the live-attenuated vaccine, including specific recommendations for its use.

Policy in the United States, as in most countries, has been aimed at preventing severe morbidity and death related to influenza; that is, preventing the complications of influenza and not influenza morbidity itself. As has been demonstrated elsewhere, the highest illness rates are experienced by children and young adults, who are less likely to experience complications and who are not now on the priority list of those to be vaccinated.

There are three levels in the US recommendations. The first is for those who should be vaccinated for their own protection, and the second is for the protection of those who can transmit virus to people in the first. The final level is a diverse listing, referred to as 'other groups to consider.' The largest group of people in level one is made up of those older than 49 years and those of any age with an underlying condition that puts them at risk of influenza complications. Vaccination recommendations based on age alone were recently lowered from age 65 years and older to include those over 49 years of age. In large part, this decision reflects the fact that 30% of people 50 to 64 years old have high-risk conditions. Vaccination rates in this group have been much lower than in those aged 65 years and older. It was decided that the most reliable way to get vaccination rates up, from a programmatic standpoint, was to recommend vaccine for the entire age group.

Table 1 lists broad groups who should receive vaccine annually for their own protection. The CDC Web site contains further details of those recommendations.[7] In addition to those older than 49 years, all residents of nursing homes or long-term facilities, regardless of age, should be vaccinated because these institutions bring together many individuals with chronic conditions. The chronic conditions for which vaccination is an absolute recommendation begin with diseases of the cardiac and pulmonary system, including asthma in persons of all ages. Diabetes mellitus is the most common metabolic disease. Renal dysfunction and hemoglobinopathies have been part of the recommendations for many years.

Immunosuppressed individuals are included in the first level of vaccine recommendations, except for individuals with human immunodeficiency virus (HIV), who are included in the category of other groups to consider. If immunosuppression is severe, antibody response may be poor and antivirals may be necessary to ensure protection. The recommendation for pregnant women is relatively new. The previous recommendation restricted vaccination to women in their second or third trimester. The association of aspirin and influenza with Reye's syndrome was documented many years ago in children and teenagers. Whenever children and teenagers require aspirin therapy, for certain forms of arthritis, for example, they should be vaccinated to prevent influenza. A new recommendation for the 2005 season recognized that there is an increased risk of hospitalization in children younger than 2 years of age and recommended vaccinating all children, age 6 months to 23 months annually. In 2005, the ACIP began recommending that those with any condition that compromises respiratory function or the handling of respiratory secretions, or that can increase the risk for aspiration (eg, those with cognitive dysfunction, spinal cord injuries, seizure disorders, or other neuromuscular disorders) be vaccinated. This recommendation in part derived from deaths of children with neuromuscular problems who died in the 2003-2004 season.

The second level involves healthy individuals who are in contact with those in need of vaccination. This is partly a recognition of the fact that in some populations, especially the frail elderly, vaccine is less efficacious than the 70% to 90% expected in healthy adults. Various categories of health-care workers who, unless protected by vaccination, can introduce infection to people who might not otherwise be exposed are in this level. A special, although similar, situation applies to families with high-risk members. Healthy family members, who are likely to be infected through contact with other people, should be vaccinated to protect the high-risk member. This particularly applies to families of children under 6 months of age. ACIP recommendations emphasize that all health-care workers should receive yearly vaccinations against influenza and strongly encourage facilities that employ health-care workers to provide vaccine to workers, using approaches designed to maximize immunization rates.

The phrase 'other group to consider' is used in ACIP recommendations to indicate groups for which vaccine can be used on a discretionary basis. These include individuals with HIV infection, who fall into this level because of questions concerning their added risk from influenza infection. Vaccination of groups such as travelers and persons providing community services will be of value to the vaccinated individuals and to the communities they visit. The ACIP recommendations also include a statement that persons in the general population who wish to prevent influenza may be vaccinated. This indicates that vaccine may be used by nearly everyone for health benefits.[7] The increased risk of hospitalization includes those under 6 months of age, but vaccination is not possible in the very young. This has now been extended to children under 5 years of age.

Evidence Supporting the ACIP Recommendations

Inactivated vaccine was developed by the US military in the 1940s to prevent what was considered a threat to military readiness. However, aside from the special populations described above, vaccine has not generally been used in healthy adults, the group in which efficacy was determined. Rather, because of the severe morbidity and mortality caused by influenza in the elderly and those with underlying conditions, vaccine was originally recommended for use in such groups in the absence of direct evaluations of effectiveness.[1] At the same time, reports of vaccine failure, especially in nursing home populations, continued to appear. As a result, despite documented cost-effectiveness, vaccination in the United States was not covered for reimbursement by Medicare in 1988. In order to include influenza vaccine as a covered benefit, Congress required studies specifically carried out in an elderly population. However, vaccine was already recommended for those

Table 2: Summary Effectiveness for Inactivated Vaccine in Preventing Pneumonia and Influenza Hospitalization, Southern Michigan

Year	Predomin-ant virus	Effectiveness in peak season (95% CI)	Effectiveness in low season
1989-90	A(H3N2) (100%)	45% (15%-64%) $P = 0.009$	21% $P = 0.4$
1990-91	B (82%)	31% (4%-51%) $P = 0.026$	2% $P = 0.9$
1991-92	A(H3N2) (80%)	32% (7%-50%) $P = 0.016$	-10% $P = 0.5$

CI = confidence interval
Adapted from Foster et al, *Am J Epidemiol* 1992;136:296-307 and from Ohmit, *Int J Epidemiol* 1995;24:1240-1248.

older than 64 years, and a trial involving placebo could not be conducted. A series of observational studies was conducted instead, which resolved the controversy. The end point in all these studies was hospitalization, a major expense for the health-care system. One study, conducted in seven counties in Michigan, examined the relationship between influenza vaccination status and hospitalization for a range of diagnoses used nationally and termed 'pneumonia and influenza' (P&I). All independently living persons older than 64 years were eligible to be included as cases and controls. Results were adjusted to control for the fact that the individuals themselves decided whether to be vaccinated. These adjustments were necessary in a nonrandomized study because although all persons in this age group were supposed to be vaccinated, those with chronic cardiopulmonary disease were more likely to be vaccinated than those without underlying conditions. Individuals with chronic illnesses were also more likely to be hospitalized. This confounding was controlled for by multivariate logistic regression analysis. Results for 3 years are shown in Table 2.[8,9]

The analyses in each year were carried out for two periods, one in which there was peak virus transmission and one in which there was little transmission, as in 1989-1990, or no transmission, as in 1990-1991 and 1991-1992. The adjustment procedures, if done properly, would be expected to demonstrate protective effectiveness during the time when influenza was circulating and little or no effectiveness at other times. It should be remembered that the outcome measure here is P&I, not laboratory-diagnosed influenza, and that even in the influenza season, there are other causes of pneumonia, which would be equal in the vaccinated and unvaccinated groups. Thus, the observed effectiveness shown in Table 2 will be less than that seen in a randomized trial when influenza infection is confirmed by laboratory means. However, the effectiveness results can be directly translated into determination of the cost savings that result during a defined period when vaccine is used. The effectiveness in the peak influenza season in preventing P&I hospitalizations was 45% during the severe 1989-1990 season and 31% in the mixed 1991-1992 year. Of particular importance is the 1990-1991 year, in which type B influenza virus predominated. The Office of Technology Assessment, in confirming the cost-effectiveness of influenza vaccine in older individuals, had assumed that vaccine would not be of value in a type B year, but this and other observations show that vaccine is effective in these seasons as well.

A similar study was conducted in Canada and was restricted to 2 A(H3N2) years.[10] The efficacies were similar to those demonstrated in Michigan, but were seen not only for P&I as the outcome, but also for other respiratory causes

Table 3: Effectiveness of Influenza Vaccination in Preventing Death Defined by Vital Statistics, Manitoba, Canada

Conditions	Outbreak Period	No. of Matched Sets
All respiratory conditions	1982-1983	155
	1985-1986	123
All causes	1982-1983	1,744
	1985-1986	1,529

Adapted from Fedson et al, *JAMA* 1993;270:1956-1961.

of hospitalization. Of particular importance in this study is that effectiveness was similar in individuals aged 45 years and older and those aged 65 years and older. In 1982-1983, 30% of cases were in the age group of 45 to 64 years, and in 1985-1986, 25% of cases were in this age group. These data would support use of vaccine in the age group younger than 65 years, in terms of clinical effectiveness. Finally, this study, because of linked records, showed effects on mortality. As shown in Table 3, vaccine in a type A(H3N2) year prevented death; this was statistically significant only for all-cause mortality because this group was larger, but the point estimate for effectiveness was higher for all respiratory conditions. This demonstrates that vaccine can prevent death as well as hospitalization.

A Minneapolis study used a different approach, working with records from a managed care organization. This method allowed investigators to follow the entire group of older individuals and did not require a case-control design, used in prior investigations.[11] Results of the

Effectiveness %	95% Confidence Interval
36	-45 to 72
50	-30 to 81
27	7 to 42
30	12 to 43

initial 3 years of this investigation identified vaccine effectiveness to be at least as good as in the Canada study, with protection as high as 57%. Of particular interest is the fact that congestive heart failure was also prevented in certain years. This finding confirmed what has been suspected for several years: that while P&I is a specific indicator of the impact of influenza, it underestimates the true impact in terms of hospitalization and death. Thus, we can expect that vaccine will also prevent events that would not have pneumonia or influenza identified as one of the diagnoses. Taken together, these and other studies confirm that influenza vaccine prevents costly events in older individuals.

Data have not been systematically collected on younger individuals with risk conditions, but as shown in Table 3, the Manitoba study suggests that vaccine should also be effective in this group. Evidence suggests that these individuals should mount a good immune response, unlike the oldest of the elderly living in nursing homes.

Nursing Home Studies

Outbreaks of influenza occur in nursing homes with high vaccination rates even when the vaccine virus is close in makeup to the circulating virus. Vaccine efficacy in nursing homes cannot be studied by randomized methods, since denying vaccine and giving placebo would not be ethical. A study conducted in Michigan by Patriarca et al showed that while vaccine was effective in nursing home residents, it was not as effective in preventing simple influenza illness as in preventing pneumonia. Death was also prevented.[12]

More recent studies have confirmed that influenza-like illness is prevented in nursing homes with influenza transmission.[13] Among the institutionalized elderly, vaccine appears to be more effective in preventing illness in younger residents. Half of the residents in these homes are younger than 85 years, and half are older. Age probably functions here as a surrogate for immune senescence, or aging of the immune system.[14]

Outbreaks of influenza in nursing homes are most frequent when A(H3N2) viruses are circulating. In 1989, a severe type A(H3N2) year, out of 45 nursing homes under study in Michigan, more than 50% of homes in which less than 80% of residents were vaccinated experienced influenza outbreaks. However, 20% of homes in which at least 80% of residents were vaccinated also had outbreaks.[15] Recent data suggest that vaccination levels above 80% still do not prevent outbreaks and indicate need for an improved vaccine, particularly for the frail elderly. Therefore, when institutionalized outbreaks of influenza occur, antivirals should be used because they protect by a nonimmunologic mechanism.

Pregnant Women

In 2005, the ACIP added pregnant women to the list of those who should be vaccinated, and specified that vaccination can occur in any trimester. Some have advocated vaccinating pregnant women for many years, based on data from the 1957 pandemic, when there was increased mortality. Recent data from the Tennessee Medicaid population support this recommendation.[16] These data show an increase in hospitalizations from cardiopulmonary events for women late in pregnancy who have underlying conditions. They also show smaller increases in hospitalizations for women without underlying conditions, which would put them in the group requiring vaccination. These data justify the recommendation that pregnant women be vaccinated but demonstrate that those most at risk are women with underlying conditions. There is ample evidence that vaccine can be given safely to these women with no harm to mother or baby. Heinonen and colleagues conducted a study of influenza vaccination involving approximately 2,000 pregnant women. The results demonstrated no adverse fetal effects associated with influenza vaccine.[17]

Vaccination of Health-Care Workers and Others to Reduce Transmission to Vulnerable Contacts

Nursing homes are one setting in which healthy health-care workers, who can respond well to vaccine, should be vaccinated. Since residents are confined to their facility, virus is likely to be introduced by workers or visitors. Some studies have suggested that vaccination of workers may be more effective in protecting residents than vaccination of the residents themselves, who might not respond as well to vaccination. Hospital workers may also expose their patients to influenza infection in a manner similar to that demonstrated for other agents, such as respiratory syncytial virus (RSV). As mentioned previously, the ACIP recommends that all health-care workers be vaccinated annually. An extension of this recommendation involves healthy family members of individuals in the identified high-risk groups. There is little direct evidence supporting this recommendation, except for data on transmission of influenza within households. The principle behind

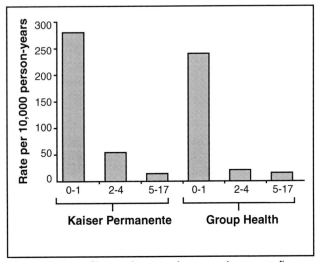

Figure 2: Rate of hospitalizations during predominant influenza seasons in non-high-risk children. Adapted from Izurieta et al, *N Engl J Med* 2000;342:232-239.

recommending vaccination of all these groups is that the healthy should respond well to vaccine.

Vaccination of Children

As previously mentioned, the ACIP recommendations for expanding vaccination have been based in large part on the principle of protecting the vaccinated, either directly by their vaccination or indirectly by vaccinating those around them. The new ACIP recommendation that children 6 months to 5 years of age be vaccinated is an example of an effort to reduce excess hospitalizations in that age group. However, children under 6 months of age are even more likely to be hospitalized, and there is no vaccine that can now be given to them. As a result, it is recommended that those around such very young children be vaccinated to protect them from exposure to infection introduced by these individuals. The concept of creating a barrier to transmission also involves others in the families of those at higher risk of complications or hospitalization, as well as health-care workers. It has been known for many years that attack rates from influenza are highest in young children; new data have shown that influenza results in hospitalization of young children, particularly those younger than 2 years. However, limitations of the inactivated vaccine, particularly the need for two injections, and the increased likelihood of adverse events with older versions of whole virus vaccine have limited vaccine use in this age group. The development of live-attenuated vaccines, which have been well tested in children younger than 5 years, has refocused attention on this issue. The FDA approved a live-attenuated vaccine (FluMist®) in 2003. It is licensed for use in healthy people between 5 and 49 years of age. See Chapter 10 for detailed information on the live-attenuated influenza vaccine (LAIV). However, assessing the impact of vaccination is complicated by the fact that influenza and RSV, a known cause of hospitalization in young children, occur in the same season. Hospitalizations of children increase during this period, but much of this increase was thought to be a result of RSV, not influenza. Evaluations of childhood hospitalization have been carried out, concentrating on years in which RSV was not a factor. Figure 2 shows the results of such analyses, focusing on two sources of data.[18] As can be seen, much of the increased hospitalization frequency occurs in children younger than 2 years, but there is also increased hospitalization in the 2- to 4-year-old age group. On this basis in 2005, ACIP began recommending annual vaccination of all children aged 6 to 23 months. This recommendation was based on data showing that children in this age group are at substantially increased risk for influenza-related hospitalization. The currently available influenza vaccines are not approved for children younger than 6 months of age.

Other Groups to Consider

While HIV infection might be considered an immuno-logic disease and therefore a listed risk factor requiring vaccine, it has also been considered as a separate group, particularly with regard to those infected who are not yet immunosuppressed. The evidence that such individuals are at increased risk of complications if infected with influenza has not been in total agreement in the past. However, it is clear that persons who are infected with HIV and have lower viral loads or $CD4^+$ counts above 100 respond well to influenza vaccine and will likely be protected.

Travelers are included as a group to consider because they may enter areas with outbreaks under way and become infected. The 2005 ACIP recommendations suggest that individuals at high risk for complications of influenza who did not receive the influenza vaccine during the preceding fall or winter should consider getting the influenza vaccine before travel if they plan to travel to the tropics, travel with organized tourist groups at any time of year, or travel to the Southern Hemisphere during April to September, when the majority of influenza activity takes place. There is no available evidence that indicates the benefits of vaccinating individuals before summer travel if they were already vac-cinated in the preceding fall. These recommendations are generally not backed by specific studies but are extensions of other recommendations and of prudent practice, such as protecting individuals providing essential community services.

Vaccination of healthy adults is a topic that has been examined extensively in recent years, with conflicting re-sults. ACIP recommendations for 2005 advise physicians that they should administer vaccine to any person who wishes to reduce the risk of becoming ill with influenza or of transmitting influenza to vulnerable individuals should they become infected. Individuals who provide essential community services should also be considered for vaccina-tion. In addition, students or others in institutional settings (eg, people living in dormitories) should be encouraged to receive vaccine. There is no doubt that influenza vaccine in healthy adults has positive health benefits; the original studies in military recruits demonstrated the protective efficacy of vaccine to be 70% to 90%. It is the cost-effectiveness of vaccination that is at issue. Recent analyses of observed data and modeling approaches have clarified some of the reasons for differences in results. The most important determinant of cost effectiveness is the size of the outbreak, which cannot be predicted in advance. If the outbreak is small, then the cost of vaccination outweighs the savings. The exact break-even point has differed in different analyses.[7] In a basically healthy population, most of the benefits are considered to be indirect; that is, not related to costs of medical care. Indirect savings are mainly derived from preventing absence from work, and the higher the pay of the individual, the greater the savings. Another issue, not easily studied, is the sustainability of programs involving a vaccine that must be administered annually and by injection. The availability of new vaccines may make this controversial area into one in which annual vaccination becomes more clearly desirable.

Thus, influenza vaccination is efficacious in all populations, but the exact protective effect may vary from group to group. Cost effectiveness has also varied somewhat from group to group, and here, economic systems need to be considered. The recommendations from ACIP have generally been evidence based; extending influenza vaccination down to age 50 years was also based on programmatic considerations. The ACIP recommendations from the United States, along with those from other countries, can be used as a guide to a rational policy for influenza vaccine use worldwide.

Vaccine Dosages and Side Effects

All influenza vaccines available in the United States can be treated as similar in their characteristics. However,

Fluzone® can be given down to age 6 months, while Fluvirin® has not been approved for use in children younger than 4 years.[19] Fluarix® can only be given to those 18 years of age or older.

Influenza vaccine should be administered by the intramuscular route. Adults and older children should be inoculated in the deltoid muscle. A needle ≥1 inch long should be used to penetrate the muscle. Infants and young children should be vaccinated in the anterolateral aspect of the thigh. Vaccine should not be given to persons with anaphylactic hypersensitivity to eggs or to those with an acute febrile illness. Children younger than 9 years should receive two doses of vaccine in the first year they are vaccinated and one dose per year thereafter. Children 6 to 35 months should receive 0.25 mL each time, and those 3 to 8 years should receive 0.5 mL each time. The adult dose of 0.5 mL should be given to those aged 9 years and older.

Minor side effects such as soreness at the inoculation site are common. More severe side effects are not often seen, although fever, malaise, myalgia, and other similar complaints have been observed, especially in children not previously vaccinated. In some recent trials in adults, there have been no differences in side effects between vaccination and placebo. A concern, since it was observed in the swine influenza experience in 1976, is Guillain-Barré syndrome. However, there has been no significant association of cases of Guillain-Barré syndrome with influenza vaccine in recent years. As with any vaccine, precautions should be taken for the possible occurrence of postvaccination anaphylaxis.

Maintaining an Adequate Vaccine Supply

In response to a serious flu vaccine shortage experienced in the United States in 2004, the FDA used its 'accelerated approval process' to obtain and evaluate the data required to license a new influenza vaccine for use in the 2005-2006 flu season. Fluarix® is approved to immunize adults 18 years of age and older against the three influenza virus A and B strains that are contained in the vaccine.

Fluarix® was the first vaccine approved using the accelerated approval process, which allows products for treating serious or life-threatening illnesses to be approved based on successfully achieving an endpoint that is reasonably likely to predict ultimate clinical benefit. Accelerated approval is usually reserved for a treatment that can be studied in a shorter period of time than is normally required for showing protection against disease. However, the manufacturer was able to demonstrate that adults who had been vaccinated with Fluarix® made levels of protective antibodies in the blood that the FDA believed were likely to be effective in preventing the flu. As a requirement of the accelerated approval, further clinical studies will be conducted to verify the clinical benefits of Fluarix®.

Universal Vaccination

It has been estimated that approximately half, or more, of all Americans are somewhere on the list of those who should be vaccinated. Many are not even aware of this situation, and it has been demonstrated that vaccination programs work best when groups are clearly delineated, such as by age. For these reasons, there has recently been an increased interest in considering universal vaccination, which would require that everyone be vaccinated on a yearly basis. It is likely that this recommendation will be implemented gradually, as more vaccine becomes increasingly available. This is one of the reasons that vaccine use has been extended to children 2-5 years of age. The rationale for vaccinating all children, especially school-age children, is strengthened by those studies suggesting that protecting school-age children will help reduce transmission in the community as a whole. Evidence for this approach is presented in Chapter 10.

References

1. Francis T Jr: The development of the 1943 vaccination study of the Commission on Influenza. *Am J Hyg* 1945;42:1-11.

2. Davenport FM: Control of influenza. *Med J Aust* 1973;suppl: 33-38.

3. Reimer CB, Baker RS, Newlin TE, et al: Influenza virus purification with the zonal ultracentrifuge. *Science* 1966;152:1379-1381.

4. Davenport FM, Rott R, Schafer, W: Physical and biological properties of influenza virus components obtained after ether treatment. *Fed Proc* 1959;18:563.

5. Wright PF, Thompson J, Vaughn WK, et al: Trials of influenza A/New Jersey/76 virus vaccine in normal children: an overview of age-related antigenicity and reactogenicity. *J Infect Dis* 1977; 136:S731-S741.

6. Wood JM, Seagroatt V, Schild GC, et al: International collaborative study of single-radial-diffusion and immunoelectrophoresis techniques for the assay of haemagglutinin antigen of influenza virus. *J Biol Stand* 1981;9:317-330.

7. Bridges CB, Thompson WW, Meltzer MI, et al: Effectiveness and cost-benefit of influenza vaccination of healthy working adults: a randomized controlled trial. *JAMA* 2000;284:1655-1663.

8. Foster DA, Talsma A, Furumoto-Dawson A, et al: Influenza vaccine effectiveness in preventing hospitalization for pneumonia in the elderly. *Am J Epidemiol* 1992;136:296-307.

9. Ohmit SE, Monto AS: Influenza vaccine effectiveness in preventing hospitalization among the elderly during influenza type A and type B seasons. *Int J Epidemiol* 1995;24:1240-1248.

10. Fedson DS, Wajda A, Nicol JP, et al: Clinical effectiveness of influenza vaccination in Manitoba. *JAMA* 1993;270:1956-1961.

11. Nichol KL, Margolis KL, Wuorenma J, et al: The efficacy and cost effectiveness of vaccination against influenza among elderly persons living in the community. *N Engl J Med* 1994;331:778-784.

12. Patriarca PA, Weber JA, Parker RA, et al: Efficacy of influenza vaccine in nursing homes. Reduction in illness and complications during an influenza A (H3N2) epidemic. *JAMA* 1985;253: 1136-1139.

13. Monto AS, Hornbuckle K, Ohmit SE: Influenza vaccine effectiveness among elderly nursing home residents: a cohort study. *Am J Epidemiol* 2001;154:155-160.

14. Ohmit SE, Arden NH, Monto AS: Effectiveness of inactivated influenza vaccine among nursing home residents during an influenza type A (H3N2) epidemic. *J Am Geriatr Soc* 1999;47:165-171.

15. Arden N, Monto AS, Ohmit SE: Vaccine use and the risk of outbreaks in a sample of nursing homes during an influenza epidemic. *Am J Public Health* 1995;85:399-401.

16. Neuzil KM, Reed GW, Mitchel EF, et al: Impact of influenza on acute cardiopulmonary hospitalizations in pregnant women. *Am J Epidemiol* 1998;148:1094-1102.

17. Heinonen OP, Shapiro S, Monson RR, et al: Immunization during pregnancy against poliomyelitis and influenza in relation to childhood malignancy. *Int J Epidemiol* 1973;2:229-235.

18. Izurieta HS, Thompson WW, Kramarz P, et al: Influenza and the rates of hospitalization for respiratory disease among infants and young children. *N Engl J Med* 2000;342:232-239.

19. Centers for Disease Control and Prevention. Prevention and control of influenza: recommendations of the Advisory Committee on Immunization Practices. *MMWR* 2002;51(RR03):1-31.

9

Chapter **10**

Influenza Prevention: Other Vaccines

Live-Attenuated Influenza Vaccines

The inactivated influenza vaccines have been available and used for almost 60 years. As indicated previously, these vaccines are effective in preventing illness and complications. However, it has been recognized for many years that improvements in vaccines for influenza would be desirable. Ideal characteristics for a new vaccine would be longer duration of immunity, greater breadth of immunity (ie, efficacy despite year-to-year changes in the virus), greater levels of protection, and a different mode of delivery. In 2003, the FDA licensed for use in the US the first vaccine using live-attenuated viruses. This live-attenuated influenza vaccine (LAIV), which is manufactured by MedImmune, Inc. and marketed under the name FluMist®, is approved for use in healthy individuals between the ages of 5 and 49. Such vaccines have been licensed and used extensively in the former Soviet Union. One of the principal advantages of live-attenuated vaccine is that it can be delivered intranasally, as a spray, rather than by parenteral injection. Other characteristics of LAIVs include the following.

• They are attenuated, producing mild or no signs or symptoms related to influenza virus infections.

• They are temperature sensitive, which limits the replication of the vaccine viruses at 38° C to 39° C, and, therefore, restricts the LAIV viruses from replicating efficiently in human lower airways.

- They are cold adapted, allowing them to replicate efficiently at 25° C, a temperature that permits the replication of LAIV viruses, but restricts the replication of different wild-type viruses.

As with the inactivated vaccines, two type A subtypes, A(H3N2) and A(H1N1), and a type B virus must be present in the live-attenuated vaccine. In addition, the exact representatives of each subtype must resemble those that are expected to circulate in the subsequent season. The selection of viruses is similar to that used for inactivated vaccines, based on the US Food and Drug Administration's and/or the World Health Organization's (WHO) recommendations. However, the requirement for updating the live-attenuated vaccine annually is different than the method used for updating the inactivated vaccine, in which the new viruses are simply substituted for the old. The attenuation of a type A and a type B influenza virus was carried out many years ago by growing them at suboptimal conditions; that is, at a reduced temperature, thus the designation of the viruses as 'cold adapted.' This produced mutations in various parts of the genome of the viruses, which rendered them able to still infect but not to cause influenza disease. The genomic changes needed to be multiple; otherwise, by back mutation, the virus could revert to virulence as it multiplied in the host. The attenuated, so-called master strains were prepared in the 1960s. The problem, then, is how to make, for example, A/Ann Arbor/6/60(H2N2), one of the master strains, induce antibodies to the contemporary type A influenza viruses.

The method used takes advantage of the segmented genome of the influenza virus, with each segment coding for a particular virion protein (see Chapter 3). For protection, antibodies to the contemporary surface antigens, hemagglutinin and neuraminidase, are necessary, and the gene segments that code for these glycoproteins in the master strain are replaced by gene segments that code for the current surface glycoproteins. The traditional way of accomplishing this is through cocultivation of the master strain with the contemporary virus. In order to select for the desired product, antibodies are used to suppress the virus carrying the old hemagglutinin and neuraminidase. The result is an attenuated virus that bears genes coding for the surface antigens of the current virus and all six internal genes of the attenuated parents. Thus, the virus used in the vaccine has the characteristics already determined by the donor parent, but still has the ability to produce the antibodies necessary for protection during the next influenza season. Because A(H3N2), A(H1N1), and B viruses must be present in the vaccine, the 'master' A virus is used twice to produce the two A subtypes, and the B donor strains are used to produce the relevant B strain. The process of selecting the contemporary viruses to be used is described in Chapter 9. The same or similar viruses are used in the live-attenuated vaccines. Variation in the exact strain used may vary depending on the availability of an appropriate virus for use in a live vaccine as well as on the growth characteristics of that virus. The WHO recommendation is stated in terms that allow flexibility in the exact strains used, as long as they have the appropriate antigenic characteristics. The live-attenuated vaccine is currently produced in pathogen-free eggs so that any adventitious agents can be excluded. This is necessary because of the lack of an inactivation step. The viruses used must similarly have been isolated and passed in only vaccine-acceptable substrates (Table 1).

American and Russian Live-Attenuated Vaccines

The American and Russian vaccines use different master strains. Both have been characterized molecularly, and the changes in the segments conferring attenuation have been determined.[1] The three circulating types and subtypes, A(H3N2), A(H1N1), and B, must be present in the vaccine. A problem in producing protection with all three viruses that does not occur with inactivated vaccines is interfer-

Table 1: Major Differences Between LAIV and Inactivated-Influenza Vaccine

Live-Attenuated Influenza Vaccine	Inactivated-Influenza Vaccine
Contains live-attenuated viruses that are still able to replicate	Contains killed viruses
Administered intranasally by sprayer	Administered intramuscularly by injection
Approved for use among healthy persons aged 5 to 49	Approved for use among persons older than 6 months including both those who are healthy and those with chronic medical conditions
More expensive than inactivated vaccine	Price differential is decreasing as of 2005

10

ence, which means that the multiplication of one virus interferes with the growth of another type or subtype. This can be partially handled by manipulating the dose used. In the American vaccine, the A(H1N1) component has not replicated as well as the other two components, and its titer has been increased to compensate. However, for those with little prior immunity (ie, young children) two inoculations have been recommended in the first year of use.

The American vaccine was evaluated in large trials using contemporary standards. In the pivotal study of the American vaccine, it was tested in children between 15 months and 71 months of age, with the median age of 43 months.[2] Most children were given two doses of vaccine, and results will be discussed for that group. The number of children

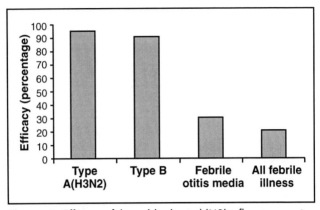

Figure 1: Efficacy of the cold-adapted (US) influenza vaccine in preventing influenza and complications in children between 15 months and 71 months of age, 1996-1997. Adapted from Belshe et al, *N Engl J Med* 1998;338:1405-1412.

given one dose was too small for definitive conclusions to be drawn, but the results did not appear to differ from those in children given the planned number of doses. Figure 1 shows the summarized results of the study. Two types of influenza were circulating during this season, 1996-1997. The efficacy of the vaccine against type A(H3N2), the more commonly identified virus, was 95%; against type B, the efficacy was 91%. When both types were combined, the resulting protective efficacy was 93%. These high efficacies have rarely been seen with inactivated vaccines evaluated using similar end points in adults.[3] However, no such comprehensive trial has ever been conducted with an inactivated vaccine in children. Without such a study, it is impossible to say that an inactivated vaccine would not have produced equally impressive results. However, this live-attenuated vaccine has demonstrated a considerable ability to prevent culture-proven influenza infection in young children.

Additional important outcomes were also evaluated. Acute otitis media is one of the most common cases of medical contact among young children, and antibiotics are frequently prescribed empirically. Information that indicates that viruses have a role in triggering acute episodes is gradually accumulating. During the course of the influenza outbreak, febrile otitis media was reduced by 30% in vaccinated children. In addition, there was a 21% reduction in total febrile illnesses over the period of the influenza outbreak.

The study of the American vaccine lasted two years. In the second year, the randomization was maintained so that children who were given vaccine in the first year were given vaccine in the second and placebo recipients received placebo again.[4] As in the first year, the exact strains used in the live vaccine were similar or identical to those used in the inactivated vaccine, based on the annual recommendation. In this year, 1997-1998, the type A(H3N2) vaccine strain was A/Wuhan/359/95(H3N2); however, in this year, the outbreak was caused by a significantly different variant, A/Sydney/5/97(H3N2). Only one inoculation was given to each child. The vaccine was found to be 86% efficacious in preventing laboratory-confirmed A/Sydney illness in the vaccinated children compared with the placebo children; 85% of those who had participated in the first year remained for the second so that there could not be a question of self-selection to continued participation of only those most medically aware. The 86% efficacy rate of the live vaccine was much higher than the efficacy of the inactivated vaccine in this year because of the antigenic difference between the A/Wuhan contained in the vaccine and the circulating A/Sydney virus. Again, the frequency of febrile influenza-like illnesses was reduced in study participants throughout the outbreak.

Following the first dose in the first year, there was a significant association of short-term rhinorrhea, nasal congestion, and low-grade fever with the vaccine. This was not seen with the second dose or in the second year, which suggests that the side effects were related to viral replication in children who would have been susceptible to infection because of little past experience with the particular virus. Again, it is impossible to say that the inactivated vaccine would not have protected at such high levels against a drifted strain in young children vaccinated for two sequential years, but that seems unlikely, based on historic and contemporary evidence.

Past studies of the American cold-adapted vaccine in adults have not shown as dramatic a difference in efficacy compared with the inactivated vaccine as that suggested by the recent results in children, even in years when the match between the circulating virus and the virus in the vaccine was good.[5] However, the first large-scale evaluation of the live influenza vaccine in adults took place in the year that A/Sydney first circulated.[6] There were 4,561 participants between the ages of 18 and 64 years. The trial was double blind and randomized, but viral end points were not identified. Only one dose of intranasal vaccine was used, and the vaccine contained the older variant A/Wuhan/395/95(H3N2). When this variant was used in the inactivated vaccine, it was not effective against the A/Sydney strain.

Several outcomes were used, but none of them involved definite influenza identification. In a year in which the inactivated vaccine was not effective, many of the reductions in occurrences in those vaccinated with the live vaccine were statistically significant. Although there was no significant difference in the prevention of all febrile illnesses, a 19% to 24% reduction was shown when the outcome was limited to severe febrile illnesses and febrile upper respiratory illnesses. The effect of vaccination on the number of days lost because of illness was also analyzed. Days with febrile illness were reduced in the vaccinated by 23%, while respiratory illness days were reduced by 41%. All of these differences were statistically significant.

When comparing these results with the preventive efficacy of approximately 90% in the childhood studies, the results in the adult studies seem low. However, it must be remembered that the adult study identified not laboratory-confirmed influenza but, instead, any illness of a particular characteristic. Even during an influenza outbreak, other illnesses occur, and, because they are not prevented by the influenza vaccine, they might have affected the results. It is clear, however, that, like the situation in children, the live vaccine protected adults in a year when the circulating virus drifted significantly from the one included in the vaccines.

Studies of the attenuated vaccine in older individuals have not been as encouraging. Many already have the antibodies to the viruses in their respiratory passages, but the antibodies do not appear to replicate reliably enough to be used without an inactivated vaccine. In a small study, it has been shown that combining the two vaccines gave better protection than the inactivated vaccine alone. Further studies are needed to determine if this would be a productive and cost-effective approach in comparison with other vaccines being developed for older individuals.[7]

Other Evidence for the Value of Live-Attenuated Influenza Vaccine

The Russian live-attenuated influenza vaccine has been used in the former Soviet Union as a licensed product for many years, and much of the work on efficacy was carried out under older standards. Also, until the last decade, results had been published in non-English-language journals. For decades, the vaccine has been used extensively for prophylaxis in children. Similar to its American counterpart, it is based on the reassortment of circulating virulent viruses with master strains that were cultivated by growth at reduced temperatures. These master strains have been defined molecularly in terms of lesions in the genome; therefore, the Russian vaccine may be considered similar enough to the US vaccine that findings from studies of the Russian vaccine can be generalized into data relevant to the class of all live influenza vaccines. Also, because the Russian vaccine is a licensed product, it has been studied under conditions of actual use.

As described elsewhere, there is evidence that schoolchildren are involved in spreading influenza in the community. Therefore, for many years, vaccination of schoolchildren has been viewed as a potential way of reducing the occurrence of influenza in the entire community. A special situation developed at the beginning of the type A(H3N2) pandemic in 1968, when a monovalent vaccine was the only vaccine available. Inactivated vaccine was used to vaccinate approximately 86% of the school-aged children, including 93% of the elementary-school-aged children, in the small community of Tecumseh, Michigan.[8] The vaccine was experimental and was unavailable for anyone else in the community or in the neighboring community of Adrian. The vaccine reduced the influenza attack rate to two thirds of that seen in Adrian. Confirmation of the validity of this approach has been derived from epidemic-modeling studies; however, use of the childhood vaccination approach for community control has not been attempted, mostly because of the need for annual vaccinations involving injections. Live vaccination with intranasal inoculation is likely to be more acceptable for regular use in community control.

The Russian live, activated vaccine was evaluated in large-scale use in schoolchildren of the city of Novgorod.[9] This live vaccine was compared with the Russian inactivated vaccine and with placebo. Each school was assigned, as a whole, to one of the two vaccines or to placebo. As a result, overall reduction in transmission could be related to a particular intervention. Thirty-four schools were involved, and children between the ages of 7 and 14 years were given one of the vaccines or placebo. However, only children whose parents agreed to their participation were inoculated, and that proportion varied from school to school. In addition, the teachers were not vaccinated and, therefore, were unprotected. The study was conducted for 2 years, one in which A(H3N2) viruses were predominant and one in which type B and type A(H1N1) viruses cocirculated. On an individual level, both the live-attenuated vaccine and the inactivated vaccine were significantly protective against respiratory illness during the defined influenza seasons. However, this did not indicate whether there was an indirect effect on reducing transmission to the unvaccinated who came in contact with the vaccinated. This was evaluated in the first year of the study by examining the effect of vaccination on the unvaccinated children and the teachers in the schools in which a varying number of students received the live vaccine, the inactivated vaccine, or placebo. In schools in which the live vaccine was used, as the percentage of the schoolchildren who were vaccinated increased, the frequency of illness in the unvaccinated children and teachers decreased, and this was statistically significant. There was no such relationship demonstrated for inactivated vaccines or, of course, for placebo. Such results could indicate that the Russian live influenza vaccine indirectly protected the unvaccinated individuals in the environment of the vaccinated individuals by reducing transmission. The fact that the inactivated vaccine did not produce indirect protection, as it did in the Tecumseh, MI, study, may relate to the fact that a higher percentage of vaccinated individuals, not achieved in Novgorod, is required for the inactivated vaccine to work in this way.

Other Live Vaccine Approaches

Additional methods are being investigated for the development and production of live virus vaccines. One, which should produce a vaccine similar to the one described above, involves the use of a process termed 'reverse genetics.'[10] Master strains known to be attenuated are used, but genes that code for the current hemagglutinin and neuraminidase are inserted by a cloning process instead of reassortment. There would have to be assurance that no mutations in the necessary surface antigens occur when the new vaccine strains are created. Another approach involves use of an entirely different live parent virus, one which is designed to not be virulent by deleting or changing some function of the virus. A deletion in the NS1 coding gene results in a virus that is more sensitive to interferon and, thus, is nonpathogenic.[11] Characteristics of such a virus would need to be evaluated in animals and in humans, especially because of the known satisfactory characteristics of the cold-adapted vaccines.

Uses of Live-Attenuated Vaccines

As mentioned previously, LAIV is an option for vaccinating healthy individuals aged 5 to 49 years. This includes healthcare workers and other individuals in close contact with people who are at high risk and those who want to avoid influenza. The possible advantages of LAIV include its ease of administration, the acceptability of the intranasal administration route over intramuscular administration, and its potential to induce a broad mucosal and systemic immune response. In their 2005-2006 recommendations, the ACIP suggested that the use of LAIV be encouraged for eligible individuals (including healthcare workers) during periods when inactivated vaccine is in short supply.

According to 2005-2006 ACIP recommendations, the following individuals should *not* be vaccinated with LAIV.
- Persons younger than 5 years or older than 50 years
- Persons with asthma, reactive airways disease, or other chronic disorders of the pulmonary or cardiovascular systems
- Persons with other underlying medical conditions, including such metabolic diseases as diabetes, renal dysfunction, and hemoglobinopathies
- Persons with known or suspected immunodeficiency diseases or who are receiving immunosuppressive therapies

- Children or adolescents receiving aspirin or other salicylates
- Persons with a history of Guillain-Barré syndrome
- Pregnant women
- Persons with a history of hypersensitivity, including anaphylaxis, to any of the components of LAIV or to eggs.

Except for individuals with a history of Guillain-Barré syndrome and hypersensitivity, all those who are ineligible for LAIV should receive inactivated influenza vaccine. In addition, the ACIP recommends the use of inactivated influenza vaccine for immunizing household members, healthcare workers, and others who have close contact with severely immunosuppressed persons. The reason for this recommendations is the theoretical risk that a live, attenuated vaccine virus could be transmitted to the severely immunosuppressed person. A health-care worker who receives LAIV should refrain from contact with severely immunosuppressed patients for 7 days after receiving the vaccine. The same recommendation applies to hospital visitors who have received LAIV. The risk for acquiring vaccine viruses from the environment is unknown, but likely to be limited. However, severely immunosuppressed individuals should also not be involved in administering LAIV.

LAIV Dosage and Administration

LAIV is for intranasal administration only and should not be administered intramuscularly, intradermally, or intravenously. It must be thawed before administration. This can be accomplished either by storing it in a refrigerator at 2° C to 8° C for 24 hours or less before use, or by holding an individual sprayer in the palm of the hand until thawed. The vaccine should not be refrozen after thawing. LAIV is supplied in a prefilled, single-use sprayer that contains 0.5 mL of vaccine. Half of the total sprayer contents (approximately 0.25 mL) is sprayed into the first nostril while the recipient is sitting or standing. A dose-divider clip, which is attached to the sprayer, must be removed to administer the second half of the dose into the other nostril.

LAIV should be administered yearly according the following schedule:

- Children aged 5 to 8 years, who have never been vaccinated with either LAIV or inactivated influenza vaccine should receive two 0.5 mL doses of LAIV separated by 6 to 10 weeks.
- Children aged 5 to 8 years who have previously been vaccinated, at any time, with either LAIV or inactivated influenza vaccine should receive 1 dose of LAIV. They do not need a second dose.
- Persons aged 9 to 49 years should receive 1 dose of LAIV.

LAIV Side Effects and Adverse Reactions

Approximately 28,000 doses of the US approved LAIV were administered to about 20,000 subjects in the 20 clinical trials conducted to assess the safety of live-attenuated vaccine. A subset of these trials were randomized, placebo-controlled studies in which approximately 4,000 healthy children aged 5 to 17 years and 2,000 healthy adults, aged 18 to 49 years were vaccinated. The incidence of adverse events that could possibly complicate influenza (e.g. pneumonia, bronchitis, or CNS events) was not statistically different among LAIV and placebo recipients aged 5 to 49. Among children, the most common side effects occurring after the first dose of LAIV included runny nose or nasal congestion, headache, vomiting, fever, and myalgias. The most common side effects among adults included runny nose or nasal congestion, headache, sore throat, chills, and tiredness or weakness. No substantial new safety concerns were revealed after an early review of reports to VAERS following the distribution of about 800,000 doses of LAIV during the 2003-2004 influenza season.

Potential Other Uses for Live-Attenuated Vaccines

It has been demonstrated that vaccination of school-aged children, if extensive enough, can protect not only the children, but also others in their environment. Whether such an approach is feasible on an annual basis will be a matter of discussion, probably for some years, as experience with the vaccine accumulates. The feasibility of such use will be a prime consideration, and the cooperation of school officials may be required, based on the direct effects that the process of preventing disruptive outbreaks may have on the schools. As in all cases, attention must be paid to maintaining such programs from year to year.

There are other populations of children in whom the vaccine will probably be used. Children in day-care facilities are particularly vulnerable to the transmission of respiratory and other infections, including influenza. In children this age, the vaccine should be highly efficacious and safe, based on the studies already conducted. Similar facilities where children are brought together in conditions that facilitate transmission would also be possible sites for use of the attenuated vaccine.

The vaccine has been shown to be effective in healthy adults and to have benefits in the workplace. The precise economic benefits of annual usage of the vaccines have been under debate and will be driven by unpredictable factors, such as the size of the outbreak, and more predictable variables, such as the salary levels of those who present with illness. Both antivirals and the inactivated vaccine will be considerations for these populations. There is, as yet, no convincing data that the live-attenuated vaccine protects adults better than the inactivated vaccine, although the route of inoculation and the ability to protect against drifted strains would seem to be advantages of the live preparation.

The population of individuals between 50 and 64 years of age, now a recommended target for inactivated vaccine, is also a group in which the live vaccine might be considered. Those who are 65 years of age and older are now the group in which annual protection is most needed. However, it is not clear whether the live vaccine will protect this group as well as the inactivated vaccine does, and studies have been hampered by ethical considerations. If the inactivated vaccine is an absolute recommendation, it is difficult to withhold it and give only the live vaccine in a clinical trial. Because studies have demonstrated that the live vaccine produces added efficacy in those also given inactivated vaccine, this may be an attractive strategy in the most vulnerable individuals older than 64 years (eg, the frail elderly in nursing homes). Further studies using innovative designs may provide more information on using only the live vaccine in at least some of the older population. In general, when a vaccine is newly introduced, we are only beginning to learn the most appropriate ways to use it, and this is certainly the case with the LAIVs. A liquid formulation, which may have less stringent requirements for storage, is currently being evaluated.

Other Vaccines Under Development

A number of different approaches to new or improved vaccines are under way. Some have even been approved for use in various countries, but not in the United States. This review is not meant to be comprehensive, but rather to summarize the spectrum of approaches being examined.

The use of adjuvants for increasing the potency of antigens has been explored for almost as long as the current inactivated vaccine has been around. In fact, many of the trials conducted by the US military involved the use of oil adjuvants. It was clear that vaccines with oil adjuvants resulted in higher titers that lasted for longer periods, two desirable features. However, the problem was that these adjuvants produced local reactions, sometimes resulting in sterile abscesses. There were also concerns about long-term consequences.[12] Most recently, work has been carried out developing a vaccine using the adjuvant MF59,which is made up of squalene (a plant and fish oil), polysorbate 80, and sorbitan trioleate. There may be two principal uses of this vaccine. When the adjuvant is used with the current yearly viruses, it appears to induce higher antibody levels in the elderly. If this translates into greater protection, it would be a major advance in vaccination for this age group, in which vaccines do not always perform ideally. This vaccine has been licensed in some European countries. This adjuvant has also been evaluated with avian antigens, such as H5,[13] which otherwise performs poorly in inducing antibodies. Other adjuvants, such as alum, are also being explored for use in a pandemic situation, in order to possibly avoid the need for a booster inoculation.

Liposome presentation of antigens has also been evaluated for many years. Liposomes are lipid membrane particles that also function as antigens.[14] All of these approaches involve vaccines produced in eggs. Vaccines that are grown in cell cultures are also being developed. These vaccines would not be subject to the vagaries of egg supply and would be of particular use in pandemics, when the supply of eggs is a rate-limiting step.

Inactivated vaccine, when presented intranasally, does not reliably induce protective antibodies. For this reason, various adjuvants have been examined for use with these antigens. One vaccine was approved in Switzerland but had to be withdrawn because of apparently serious side effects; others are now under study. Intranasal delivery would make annual vaccination more acceptable.

Finally, molecular approaches are being pursued. The viral hemagglutinin can be expressed in baculovirus, an insect virus. This has been done with the H5 antigen of Hong Kong avian influenza, which was impossible to grow in eggs.[15] Unfortunately, the human response to this antigen has been less than optimal. A more general strategy for producing immune response is DNA vaccination. This method, sometimes referred to as 'naked DNA,' involves the use of a 'gene gun' for DNA-encoded antigens, would mimic live vaccination, and could be used for any protein antigen. The strategy is in its infancy, and various concerns, including efficacy and safety questions, must be addressed.

References

1. Kendal AP, Maassab HF, Alexandrova GI, et al: Development of cold-adapted recombinant live, attenuated influenza A vaccines in the USA and USSR. *Antiviral Res* 1981;1:339-365.

2. Belshe RB, Mendelman PM, Treanor J, et al: The efficacy of live attenuated, cold-adapted, trivalent, intranasal influenza virus vaccine in children. *N Engl J Med* 1998;338:1405-1412.

3. Heikkinen T, Ruuskanen O, Waris M, et al: Influenza vaccination in the prevention of acute otitis media in children. *Am J Dis Child* 1991;145:445-448.

4. Belshe RB, Gruber WC, Mendelman PM, et al: Efficacy of vaccination with live attenuated, cold-adapted, trivalent, intranasal influenza virus vaccine against a variant (A/Sydney) not contained in the vaccine. *J Pediatr* 2000;136:168-175.

5. Edwards KM, Dupont WD, Westrich MK, et al: A randomized controlled trial of cold-adapted and inactivated vaccines for the prevention of influenza A disease. *J Infect Dis* 1994;169:68-76.

6. Nichol KL, Mendelman PM, Mallon KP, et al: Effectiveness of live, attenuated intranasal influenza virus vaccine in healthy, working adults: a randomized controlled trial. *JAMA* 1999;282:137-144.

7. Treanor JJ, Mattison HR, Dumyati G, et al: Protective efficacy of combined live intranasal and inactivated influenza A virus vaccines in the elderly. *Ann Intern Med* 1992;117:625-633.

8. Monto AS, Davenport FM, Napier JA, et al: Modification of an outbreak of influenza in Tecumseh, Michigan by vaccination of school children. *J Infect Dis* 1970;122:16-25.

9. Rudenko LG, Slepushkin AN, Monto AS, et al: Efficacy of live attenuated and inactivated influenza vaccines in schoolchildren and their unvaccinated contacts in Novgorod, Russia. *J Infect Dis* 1993;168:881-887.

10. Garcia-Sastre A, Palese P: Genetic manipulation of negative-strand RNA virus genomes. *Annu Rev Microbiol* 1993;47:765-790.

11. Talon J, Salvatore M, O'Neill RE, et al: Influenza A and B viruses expressing altered NS1 proteins: a vaccine approach. *Proc Natl Acad Sci U S A* 2000;97:4309-4314.

12. Weibel RE, McLean A, Woodhour AF, et al: Ten-year follow-up study for safety of adjuvant 65 influenza vaccine in man. *Proc Soc Exp Biol Med* 1973;143:1053-1056.

13. Nicholson KG, Colegate AE, Podda A, et al: Safety and antigenicity of non-adjuvanted and MF59-adjuvanted influenza A/Duck/Singapore/97 (H5N3) vaccine: a randomised trial of two potential vaccines against H5N1 influenza. *Lancet* 2001;357:1937-1943.

14. Rimmelzwaan GF, Nieuwkoop N, Brandenburg A, et al: A randomized, double blind study in young healthy adults comparing cell mediated and humoral immune responses induced by influenza ISCOM™ vaccines and conventional vaccines. *Vaccine* 2000;19:1180-1187.

15. Treanor JJ, Wilkinson BE, Masseoud F, et al: Safety and immunogenicity of a recombinant hemagglutinin vaccine for H5 influenza in humans. *Vaccine* 2001;19:1732-1737.

10

Chapter 11

Antivirals for Influenza: The Basics

For almost 40 years, it has been recognized that influenza replication can be affected by drugs that are clinically relevant. Why then, has it taken so long to define a clear role for drugs in the prophylaxis and treatment of influenza? Influenza is no longer discounted in terms of its potential for causing severe disease. Rather, much of the problem relates to the history of the first class of drugs to be introduced, the adamantanes, more recently termed the *M2 inhibitors* based on their mechanism of action in inhibiting the replication of type A viruses. These drugs were before their time, developed before the use of antiviral drugs in general, not simply their role in influenza management, was appreciated. Unfortunately, in some quarters, this problem has continued and has led to a reluctance to value appropriate therapies that ordinarily could have been automatically accepted. Had the influenza antivirals been introduced after the antiherpes drugs, their acceptance might have been more rapid.

The first of the M2 inhibitors, amantadine (Symmetrel®), was developed in the early 1960s.[1] There is some controversy about whether its efficacy was first identified for influenza or Parkinson's disease. It was probably during the study of its effects on type A influenza that its value in control of some Parkinsonian symptoms was recognized. The drug was first licensed in 1966 specifically for type A(H2N2) influenza, and that subtype promptly ceased its transmission in 1968. It was recognized even at that time that the adamantanes were effective against all type A viruses, but it was not until 1976 that they were registered again for use against the type A(H3N2) virus, which appeared that year in a pandemic form. In fact, because it was reported that amantadine worked against the new virus at a time when little vaccine was available, it began to be used off label. The manufacturer was asked to send out a 'Dear Doctor' letter as a reminder that amantadine was not approved for use against the new subtype. Finally, registration for use against all type A viruses was approved, which helped when the type A(H1N1) virus appeared in North America in late 1978. During the hiatus, amantadine's usefulness in treating Parkinson's disease sustained its continued production.

Throughout this period, the concept of an antiviral for influenza was treated as an exotic approach to disease control. Even inactivated influenza vaccine was treated with some suspicion, with questions repeatedly raised about its safety and efficacy. The arrival of type A(H1N1) influenza in the pseudopandemic of 1978, which was limited to children and young adults, led to a change in this opinion. The change involved both prophylaxis and therapy of type A influenza. First, it was clearly demonstrated during the 1978 outbreak that amantadine was more than 70% effective in preventing symptomatic, laboratory-confirmed influenza. These observations were quickly extended to rimantadine (Flumadine®) and both subtypes of prevalent type A viruses, A(H3N2) and A(H1N1). Data also began to accumulate on therapy, although the studies remained small and clear benefit was often difficult to quantify. Throughout the 1980s and into the 1990s, the M2 inhibitors gradually gained increased acceptance for treatment and control of type A influenza.

The central nervous system activity of amantadine, which allowed the drug to survive the hiatus in licensure for influenza, meant that some patients experienced side effects such as insomnia, difficulty concentrating, and unsteadiness. This raised the issue of whether people taking amantadine might be impaired while driving. For this reason, during the 1980s and even before, many of the experimental studies organized by the National Institutes of Health involved rimantadine, the other M2 inhibitor. However, the developer of both drugs, DuPont Pharmaceuticals, did not wish to bring both drugs to the market. Therefore, rimantadine was not licensed until 1993, when it was sold to another pharmaceutical company.

Rimantadine was viewed as a major advance, and it was hoped that it would result in more extensive use of influenza antivirals. However, amantadine and rimanta-dine had significant limitations, including effect only against type A influenza and emergence of resistance when used in treatment, especially in close populations. Thus, identification and evaluation of a new class of antivirals, the neuraminidase inhibitors, which were effective against both type A and B influenza, were welcomed. This development was the ultimate result of the determination of the crystalline structure of influenza neuraminidase and the identification of sites in a portion of the virus that was similar in both type A and B viruses.[2] This computer-engineered drug design resulted in two new compounds, zanamivir (Relenza®) and oseltamivir (Tamiflu®). Drug development was different in the 1990s, and studies evaluating therapy and prophylaxis were far larger than those of the M2 inhibitors, allowing precise estimates of efficacy to be made. Resistance did not seem to be a major problem, and unlike the M2 inhibitors, treatment with the new drugs prevented complications of influenza. The characteristics of drugs of both classes are presented in detail below.

The M2 Inhibitors

The two drugs of this class, amantadine and rimantadine, are available in the United States. Only amantadine is licensed in many other countries, including Canada. While

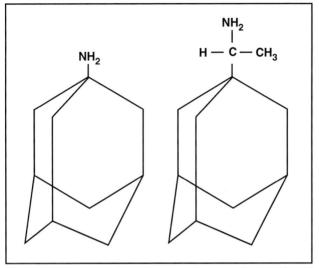

Figure 1: The chemical structures of amantadine (left) and rimantadine (right).

these drugs are similar in antiviral activity and propensity to select for resistant strains, their pharmacokinetics and safety profile are different. As indicated below, a recently detected increase in antiviral resistance has limited their utility.

Structure and Activity

Amantadine and rimantadine belong to a unique class of compounds originally described in the late 1950s and early 1960s. Their chemical structures are shown in Figure 1. They are colorless crystalline amines with an unusual symmetrical structure. Both have a large carbon ring (the adamantyl cage) and a primary amine. In amantadine, the amine is directly linked to the cage, but in rimantadine, the amine is separated by a branched side chain that provides a center of asymmetry. These differences affect their metabolism and their ability to pass the blood-brain barrier.

The name for the compounds was derived from the same origins as the word 'diamond,' based on their hardness and stability. This stability may be of use in stockpiling these drugs for use in pandemics.

Because amantadine was the first drug to be developed, its spectrum of activity was extensively studied. There were hopes that it would be active against a broad spectrum of viruses, but, although there was some in vitro reduction of viruses such as rubella, such activity was not achieved at clinically relevant concentrations.[3] The surprise, considering the imperfect understanding of viruses at that time, was that the activity of amantadine and, later, that of rimantadine, was limited to type A influenza. It did not extend to type B viruses or the more distantly related parainfluenza viruses. Thus there is no justification for use of these compounds against other viruses that have been the subject of occasional anecdotal reports. The antiviral activity of the drugs was confirmed in laboratory animals, particularly in mice and ferrets, in which an infection similar to that in humans can be produced.

For many years, the mechanism of the antiviral activity of the adamantanes was poorly understood. By contrast, the neuraminidase inhibitors were developed to interfere with a necessary component of viral replication. Paradoxically, understanding the mechanism of action of the adamantanes was assisted by the observation that resistance to them, when they were used in treatment, emerged rapidly and predictably.[4] The M2 inhibitors have a number of complex activities in inhibiting viral replication, but they principally block the M2 ion channel by which the virus is uncoated and thereby readied for further replication. Uncoating is a necessary first step that must precede viral transcription, translation, and assembly. The M2 protein serves as an acid-activated ion channel that permits protein transfer across the membrane of the virus. The drugs bind to this protein, causing a conformational change and interfering with the ion channel.[5] This interferes with the acidification of the interior of the virus so that the uncoating of the virus does not occur. The type B viruses do not possess an M2 protein, which explains the specificity of the M2 inhibitors. The importance of the M2 protein is further confirmed by the fact that resistance to the antivirals is associated with the substitution of one of several amino acids in it. These substitutions render achievable levels of either M2 inhibitor ineffective against the virus. Viruses that are resistant to one drug are resistant to the other.

Metabolism, Pharmacokinetics, and Toxicology

The similarities of amantadine and rimantadine in their resistance patterns are not carried forward in their pharmokinetics. Amantadine was recognized early as a useful drug in the treatment of Parkinson's disease. That was not the case with rimantadine, and because it was more attractive to develop a drug for two indications than for one, rimantadine was developed much later as an antiviral in the United States. The difference in the ability of the two drugs to cross the blood-brain barrier has been confirmed in animal studies, and amantadine's role in affecting the brain's extrapyramidal system is borne out by differences in side effects.

Both drugs are administered orally as hydrochloride salts, and they are well absorbed from the gastrointestinal tract.[6,7] There is no preparation available for parenteral administration. After a single oral dose of amantadine, peak plasma levels are reached in 2 to 4 hours. With rimantadine, peak levels are achieved in 3 to 6 hours. It has therefore been suggested that a loading dose be given so that adequate blood levels might be achieved more rapidly. This would seem to be an advantage in therapy, where treatment initiated earlier should result in more rapid resolution of symptoms. However, in a small trial involving rimantadine, a loading dose did not demonstrate any advantage over regular dosing. The half-life of rimantadine is 37 hours, compared with 17 hours for amantadine; however, both are long enough that single daily dosing can be considered in prophylaxis. Twice-daily dosing is now recommended. Peak levels of amantadine are nearly twice as high as those of rimantadine for the same dose, but the concentration of rimantadine in nasal mucus is about 50% higher than that of amantadine. These differences have resulted in debates on whether the drugs' activities should be compared at the same dosage, as they generally have been.

Metabolism and excretion of the two drugs are profoundly different. Amantadine is mainly excreted unchanged by renal tubular secretion. In contrast, rimantadine is extensively metabolized by the liver, with up to 90% excreted in the form of hydroxylated and conjugated metabolites, only some of which have antiviral activity. Since only 2% to 20% of amantadine is excreted unchanged, there is much more concern about accumulation with amantadine.[8] Accumulation partly explains some of the side effects seen with amantadine, especially in the frail elderly, when the level of renal dysfunction has not been recognized. Reduction of dosage with rimantadine is also recommended in persons with advanced renal and hepatic disease, but drug interactions have been more systematically evaluated with rimantadine than amantadine. In a single-dose study, plasma concentration of rimantadine was consistently but modestly higher when cimetidine (Tagamet®) was administered. This and effects seen with aspirin and acetaminophen were considered of little clinical significance.

Animal toxicity studies have not been performed for the M2 inhibitors to the same extent as they have for newer drugs. There has been evidence of moderate reduction in fertility with amantadine in rats. Failed fertility has been reported anecdotally in humans. Teratogenicity and embryolethality have been observed in rats but not in rabbits. Similar data have resulted with rimantadine. Some abnormalities in rabbit fetuses have also been observed with rimantadine.

Neuraminidase Inhibitors (NAIs): Introduction

Viral neuraminidase is essential for efficient replication of the virus. Hemagglutinin enables the virus to attach to the cell surface, and neuraminidase, also termed sialidase, is the enzyme that cleaves the attachment to the sialic acid residues on the cell surface to release it. Neuraminidase also keeps the viral particles from adhering to each other and forming clumps, which would inhibit their ability to infect new cells.[2] It may also help in breaking down the mucus barrier to allow infection of the cells of the respiratory tract. Thus, inhibiting enzymatic activity will also inhibit the replication of the virus. Early attempts at developing a neuraminidase-inhibiting drug showed that the concept was correct; however, these drugs were not specific to the influenza neuraminidase and acted on similar enzymes in, for example, the liver and the placenta.[9] Determination of the crystalline structure of the virus neuraminidase facilitated the design of the neuraminidase inhibitors.[10] It enabled researchers to design drugs that fit into the enzymatically active site of the virus, or the 'conserved' area, where the structure and amino acids are similar in both type A and B viruses. In fact, the conserved area is similar in all nine type A neuraminidases recognized in nature, particularly in avian species.[11,12] This has particular relevance regarding use of these drugs in a pandemic situation. Two neuraminidase-inhibiting drugs are licensed in the United States, and at least one other is in development. They appear to be relatively similar in their antiviral activity, even though they differ in the way they may be used.[13]

Structure and Activity of Zanamivir

The structure of zanamivir, along with that of sialic acid, is shown in Figure 2. The resemblance of zanamivir, the first NAI to be developed, to sialic acid allows the drug to compete successfully with sialic acid to fit into a pocket, or cleft, of the neuraminidase. The guanido group facilitates this attachment but prevents the drug from being

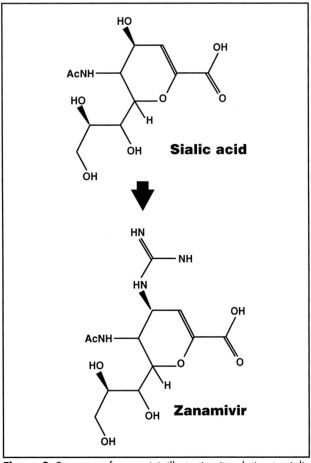

Figure 2: Structure of zanamivir illustrating its relation to sialic acid by replacement of the 4-hydroxy group with a guanido group.

well absorbed from the gastrointestinal tract. Zanamivir is therefore administered by oral inhalation as a dry powder. This method of administration is unique for an antiviral.

Zanamivir is prepared for administration as a dry powder blended with a lactose carrier. The resultant mixture contains 20 mg of lactose and 5 mg of zanamivir. This is contained in a blister that is penetrated when used in the Diskhaler® device. It is inhaled by active inspiration. No propellant is used. Two inhalations are the standard dose, giving a total of 10 mg of zanamivir. When administered in this way, the drug is deposited throughout the respiratory tract from the throat downward. Some of the drug is swallowed so that on positron emission tomography large amounts of radiolabeled zanamivir are found in the stomach.[14] However, the amount of drug deposited in the lower respiratory tract is well above that needed to inhibit replication of the influenza virus.

Antiviral activity is broad, as would be expected. The exact concentrations required to inhibit type A and B virus vary but are easily achievable in the lower respiratory tract. In animal studies, zanamivir was at least 100 times more active than amantadine. It has also been shown to be active against neuraminidases present in avian species, which may be involved in the next pandemic.

Metabolism, Excretion, and Toxicology of Zanamivir

Little of the administered drug is absorbed. This is generally not a problem because influenza is not usually a systemic infection. However, the likelihood of prevention of complications such as sinusitis may be reduced. The 15% of drug that is absorbed is eliminated unchanged by the kidneys. Renal impairment would affect this excretion. However, so little drug is absorbed that no reduction in dose is necessary in renally impaired patients. Pharmacokinetics have also been studied after intravenous administration, but no such preparation of zanamivir is available for use.

Zanamivir has been shown not to interfere with the cytochrome P450 isoenzymes. No significant drug-drug interactions have been detected, and the route of administration makes such interactions unlikely. There was a study to determine whether administration of zanamivir inhibited the response to inactivated influenza virus vaccination. No such effect was detected.

In animal toxicology studies, no carcinogenesis or mutagenesis has been observed. There was no effect of the drug on fertility or mating behavior in rats. In studies examining possible effects on fetal development in rabbits and rats, there were inconsistent effects on skeletal development. It was unclear whether these were above the background level. No formal studies in pregnant or lactating women have been carried out.

Structure and Activity of Oseltamivir

Oseltamivir is an ethyl ester prodrug that is administered orally and is rapidly converted by hepatic esterases to its active metabolite, oseltamivir carboxylate. Similar to zanamivir, oseltamivir has specific activity against the neuraminidase of influenza and not against the sialadases of parainfluenza viruses, various bacteria, or human liver microsomes. It has been found, in the laboratory and in experimental animals, to be active at clinically relevant concentrations against a wide variety of different type A and B influenza isolates and archival strains.

The structures of the prodrug and the carboxylate are shown in Figure 3. Oseltamivir is similar to zanamivir but contains a cyclohexene ring and a lipophilic side chain. It attaches to the enzymatically active site of the neuraminidase by electrostatic and hydrophobic mechanisms.

Metabolism, Pharmacokinetics, and Toxicology of Oseltamivir

Oseltamivir is rapidly absorbed from the gastrointestinal tract. Plasma concentrations of oseltamivir carboxylate are detectable within 30 minutes of an oral dose. Peak drug concentrations are reached in 3 to 4 hours. There is high oral bioavailability of close to 80% of the oral dose, indicating excellent absorption. Food does not inhibit absorption, so the drug can be administered with a meal or snack to

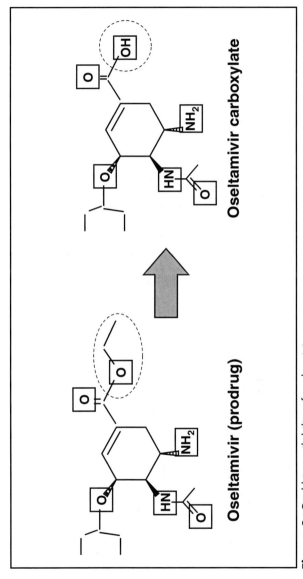

Figure 3: Oral bioavailability of oseltamivir.

11

153

reduce the possibility of gastrointestinal upset. The drug is widely distributed to sites such as the middle ear and sinuses. Concentration of the drug in bronchoalveolar fluids appears to be significantly higher than that in the blood.

Oseltamivir carboxylate is eliminated from the body through the kidneys by glomerular filtration and renal tubular secretion. Of a single oral dose of oseltamivir, 63% is eliminated as the active metabolite in the urine. A reduction in dosage is therefore recommended for patients with severe renal insufficiency (see Chapter 13). Renal clearance varies with age, but not sufficiently to require change in dosage on that basis alone.[15]

No drug-drug interactions have been demonstrated with oseltamivir and acetaminophen or amoxicillin. No competition for esterases or interactions with cimetidine have been observed. Probenecid (Probalan®) is excreted by a similar mechanism as oseltamivir, but no reduction in oseltamivir dosage is necessary when probenecid is used.

Animal toxicity studies were carried out using increasing dosages of the drug. Mutagenicity was negative in the Ames test. There were no effects on fertility, mating performance, or early embryonic developments in rats. Some minor skeletal abnormalities were seen in rats and rabbits. Studies in pregnant women have not been carried out, so it is unknown whether these findings would apply to humans. However, these side effects are clearly of much lower potential magnitude than those seen with the M2 inhibitors.

Other Antivirals for Influenza

The four influenza antivirals licensed for use in the United States inhibit influenza virus replication by targeting two different sites. Given the complexity of viral replication, other approaches in antiviral drug development have been evaluated. Blocking attachment of the virus to the host cell at the hemagglutinin level has not been particularly successful. Protease inhibitors, which have been successful in treating other viral infections, have been studied extensively. Unfortunately, none has yet had the necessary specificity. Nucleoside analogues have also been evaluated. One, ribavirin (Virazole®), has been extensively evaluated. It was found to be too toxic to be administered orally, and thus a special device was used for aerosol administration, similar to that now in use for children with respiratory syncytial virus infection. For influenza, the treatment effect was small. Combined with the difficulty in administration, this finding made ribavirin not promising enough for clinical trials to continue. The current two classes of drugs, the M2 inhibitors and the NAIs, are therefore the only choices for prophylaxis and therapy of influenza for the foreseeable future. The only additional anti-influenza drug that has been in large-scale trials is another NAI.

References

1. Davies WL, Grunert RR, Haff RF, et al: Antiviral activity of L-adamantanamine (amantadine). *Science* 1964;144:862-863.

2. Laver WG, Bischofberger N, Webster RG: Disarming flu viruses. *Sci Am* 1999;280:78-87.

3. Maassab HF, Cochran KW: Rubella virus: inhibition in vitro by amantadine hydrochloride. *Science* 1964;145:1443-1444.

4. Hay AJ: The mechanism of action of amantadine and rimantadine against influenza viruses. In: Notkins AL, Oldstone MB, eds. *Concepts in Viral Pathogenesis III*. New York, NY, Springer-Verlag, pp 561-567, 1989.

5. Sugrue RJ, Hay AJ: Structural characteristics of the M2 protein of influenza A viruses: evidence that it forms a tetrameric channel. *Virology* 1991;180:617-624.

6. Aoki FY, Sitar DS: Clinical pharmacokinetics of amantadine hydrochloride. *Clin Pharmacokinet* 1988;14:35-51.

7. Wills RJ: Update on rimantadine's clinical pharmacokinetics. *J Resp Dis* 1989;10:20-25.

8. Wu MJ, Ing TS, Soung LS, et al: Amantadine hydrochloride pharmacokinetics in patients with impaired renal function. *Clin Nephrol* 1982;17:19-23.

9. Palese P, Schulman J, Bodo G, et al: Inhibition of influenza and parainfluenza virus replication in tissue culture by 2-deoxy-2, 3-dehydro-N-trifluoroacetylneuraminic acid (FANA). *Virology* 1974;59:490-498.

10. von Itzstein I, Wu WY, Kok G, et al: Rational design of potent sialidase-based inhibitors of influenza virus replication. *Nature* 1993;363:418-423.

11. von Itzstein M, Dyason JC, Oliver SW, et al: A study of the active site of influenza virus sialidase: an approach to the rational design of novel anti-influenza drugs. *J Med Chem* 1996;39:388-391.

12. Luo M, Air GM, Brouillette WJ: Design of aromatic inhibitors of influenza virus neuraminidase. In: Brown LE, Hampson AW, Webster RG, eds. *Options for the Control of Influenza III*. Amsterdam, Elsevier, pp 702-712, 1996.

13. Gubareva LV, Kaiser L, Hayden FG: Influenza virus neuraminidase inhibitors. *Lancet* 2000;355:827-835.

14. Bergstrom M, Cass LM, Valind S, et al: Deposition and disposition of [11C] zanamivir following administration as an intranasal spray. Evaluation with positron emission tomography. *Clin Pharmacokinet* 1999;36:33-39.

15. McClellan K, Perry CM: Oseltamivir: a review of its use in influenza. *Drugs* 2001;61:263-283.

Chapter 12

M2 Inhibitors for Prevention and Treatment

The M2 inhibitors amantadine (Symmetrel®) and rimantadine (Flumadine®) are efficacious in preventing and treating type A influenza. They are ineffective against type B viruses, which is a problem when type A and B viruses occur at the same time. This situation is shown in Figure 1. The same situation was observed in 2000-2001. The data on efficacy in prophylaxis are explicit because the sample sizes were large enough to produce clear results. Also, the end point in prophylactic studies on the prevention of laboratory-confirmed clinical influenza is incontrovertible. In treatment, no agreed end point was used, and the studies were small by current standards. This does not mean that the M2 inhibitors are not efficacious in treatment; it is just difficult to draw as clear a conclusion as can be reached with the neuraminidase inhibitors. However, recent reports of high levels of antiviral resistance in global isolates has rendered these drugs of limited usefulness. (Chapter 13).

Seasonal Prophylaxis

The efficacy of an antiviral in preventing an influenza outbreak over the course of the influenza season is most simply defined as seasonal prophylaxis. Two studies of

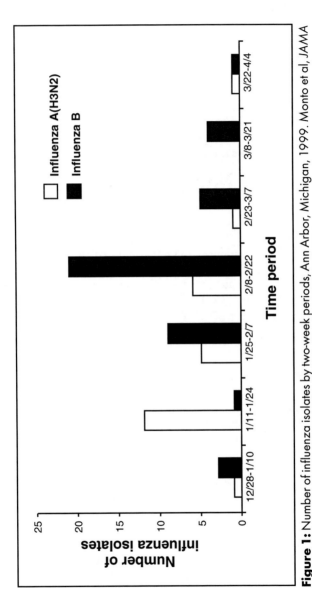

Figure 1: Number of influenza isolates by two-week periods, Ann Arbor, Michigan, 1999. Monto et al, *JAMA* 1979;241:1003-1007; Dolin et al, *N Engl J Med* 1982;307:580-584.

Table 1: Protective Efficacy of M2 Inhibitors Against Laboratory-Confirmed Clinical Influenza

Site and Subtype	Efficacy	Significance
Michigan Type A(H1N1)		
Amantadine	71%	$P < 0.001$
Vermont Types A(H3N2) and A(H1N1)		
Amantadine	91%	$P < 0.001$
Rimantadine	85%	

seasonal prophylaxis of amantadine and rimantadine were conducted in the 1970s and 1980s and established that both drugs are similarly efficacious; results are shown in Table 1. Both studies were performed over a 6-week period, after influenza transmission had been detected in the area. Outbreaks may last longer, but the peak transmission takes place during this period.

The first study, conducted in Michigan, was carried out when the type A(H1N1) virus returned in 1978 after a 20-year absence.[1] Individuals younger than 25 years had few or no antibodies to this virus. As a result, major outbreaks took place, but they were restricted to younger adults and children. This has been termed a pseudopandemic because it had rapid worldwide spread but was restricted to an age group. College campuses were particularly affected, and the study at the University of Michigan was initiated in the face of the outbreak. Differences in illness frequency between those on drug and those on placebo became significant 2 days after individuals had been put on prophylaxis. Overall, the efficacy of the drug in preventing laboratory-confirmed clinical influenza was 71%, with much of the difference in the first 2 weeks of the study (ie, the time of peak influenza transmission). Protection against all influenza infection, symptomatic and asymptomatic, detected serologically, was 40%. This indicated that the drug was more effective in preventing infections with symptoms than infections without symptoms.

The second study was carried out 3 years later, and, at that time, two prevalent type A viruses, A(H3N2) and A(H1N1), cocirculated.[2] A rimantadine arm was included; protection was equivalent at 91% for amantadine and 85% for rimantadine. The difference between the efficacy of amantadine in the first study and that in the second study could relate to the fact that M2 inhibitors seem to act together with antibodies in protecting against disease. The interpretation would be that, in the first study, no antibodies against the circulating virus were present in the population because the virus A(H1N1) was novel for the involved age group. This resulted in reduced protection compared with the protection seen in the second study, when antibodies were present; the population at that time had experience with both viruses. The overall conclusion is that the range of protection produced by the M2 inhibitors is 70% to 90%, similar to that of vaccines, and the two drugs are equivalent in producing that protection.

Side effects were assessed in both investigations. Withdrawals from the study were used in the first trial as a way of recognizing that an adverse event was of importance to the participants. The difference in the first study between the withdrawals from the group on amantadine and those from the group on placebo was 6%. In the second study, 11% of all withdrawals were attributable to amantadine, but there were no differences between withdrawals of individuals on placebo and on rimantadine. This was one of the first indications of the greater likelihood of amantadine to produce side effects. Most of these effects are related to the central nervous system, and most are mild, but they can be troublesome enough in young adults to cause withdrawal from a clinical trial.

Seasonal prophylaxis is not a practical approach for most situations, especially when a vaccine is available, matches the circulating strains, and can be used without contraindications. Antivirals need to be taken daily and may produce side effects. Targeted prophylactic approaches have been suggested instead, for use over a shorter period. For example, individuals exposed to a person with influenza may be put on short-term prophylaxis. Generally, this approach also involves treatment. Travelers who may be exposed to influenza at a time when vaccine is not available may also use targeted prophylaxis.

One population in which seasonal prophylaxis may be useful is the frail elderly living in nursing homes. Putting residents on prophylaxis when there is community transmission of type A viruses is based on the fact that outbreaks of influenza can occur in nursing homes with high vaccination rates. Nursing homes are places where individuals who may respond poorly to vaccine are brought together in settings where transmission is likely to occur if virus is introduced. Studies with the M2 inhibitors show that the drugs have a protective effect in vaccinated individuals.[3] Seasonal prophylaxis in nursing homes could be a supplement to vaccination but should never be a substitute.

12

Treatment With M2 Inhibitors

The precise effect of amantadine and rimantadine in treating cases of type A influenza is difficult to determine because studies of their use in treatment were relatively small and used different end points. A meta-analysis that concentrates on fever has been published, but fever is only one component of the influenza syndrome. It can be concluded that, as in prophylaxis, the therapeutic effect of both drugs is similar. However, in the United States, rimantadine is licensed only for treatment of adults because of a lack of sufficient data on its use in the treatment of children.

Rimantadine is approved for prophylaxis among children age 1 year and older.

All treatment studies required patients to have been ill for no more than 2 days. Therefore, it is impossible to draw conclusions about the effect of M2 inhibitor treatment in patients who present after 2 days, which is a common occurrence.

In a study in which treatment began within 2 days of illness onset, patients on drug were febrile for half as long as patients on placebo. Other studies have demonstrated more modest reductions in duration of fever and symptom scores in the treated patients compared with those given placebo.[4,5] Of particular relevance in demonstrating therapeutic effect is one study that compared amantadine to aspirin in the treatment of adults.[6] This study was performed mainly to confirm that the value of the M2 inhibitors was greater than the value of standard antipyretics. At that time, many skeptics thought that M2 inhibitors were no more than a 'super aspirin.' As in most studies, a symptom score was used to assess reduction in the severity of symptoms, of which fever was only one. Aspirin at 3.25 g daily outperformed amantadine on the first day of treatment, but the antiviral subsequently outperformed the antipyretic. This indicates the importance of antiviral therapy, which may have long-term positive effects, including shortening the duration of illness and allowing individuals to return to productive activity more quickly. The most desirable effect would be a reduction in the complications of influenza, which has never been seen with the M2 inhibitors, perhaps because of small numbers of patients or inappropriate end points. In a study of volunteers challenged with influenza and given either an M2 inhibitor or a neuraminidase inhibitor, there was a positive effect on middle-ear pressure with the latter but not with the former, which suggests a real difference between the classes of drugs. The only study that showed a positive effect of the M2 inhibitors on small airways was one conducted during an A(H3N2) outbreak. This virus is the subtype most likely to lead to complications. The small-airway abnormalities were observed in some untreated individuals, but, in treated persons, their frequency was significantly reduced.[7]

Treatment of children with the M2 inhibitors has only been studied imperfectly. Even the recommended dose of amantadine for children (4.4 to 8.8 mg/kg/day, not to exceed 150 mg/day) was empirically defined. Amantadine is the only drug licensed for the treatment of children. In one study, rimantadine, which has been approved for prophylaxis in children older than one year, was compared with acetaminophen instead of placebo. This produced little difference in outcome.[8] The most conclusive study, that of Hall et al, did show a beneficial effect of rimantadine in a study involving 69 children.[9] However, an unexpected finding was the isolation of antiviral-resistant viruses late in therapy. This did not appear to have a negative effect on therapeutic activity; recovery proceeded more rapidly in the treated group. At the time, it was treated as an interesting but not significant finding. However, it was later confirmed that many adults also shed resistant viruses, but they recover as rapidly as those who do not. More recently, with the recognition of the importance of antiviral resistance, this finding has assumed greater importance,[10] emphasized by a recent observation in Japan that suggests that the shedding of resistant viruses may be accompanied by a recrudescence of fever in some children late in the course of the illness. The return of fever in young children, but not in adults, may be caused by more pronounced virus replication and longer duration of illness in infected children, which increases the chance of the resistant viruses again producing symptoms.

Household Prophylaxis With M2 Inhibitors

The family is a common site of virus transmission, and influenza attack rates are higher in families than in the community. However, not all of what appear to be intrafamilial infections are acquired from family members because the outbreak in the community is ongoing and new introductions are possible. To reduce the attack rate in a household, once influenza has been introduced, the strategy is to treat the first, or index, case and to put the rest of the family on prophylaxis for a limited time. Before and after the 1968 A(H3N2) pandemic, Galbraith et al conducted two household-based studies.[11,12] In the first, the infecting virus was A(H2N2); the contacts were placed on prophylaxis, but the index cases were not treated. Protection against developing illness was demonstrated in the contacts. In the second study, after the A(H3N2) virus arrived, the index cases were treated and the contacts were given prophylaxis. No prophylactic efficacy was seen in the contacts. At the time, it was believed that the lack of effect was related to the fact that A(H3N2) was a new virus for the entire population and that, without 'help' from a specific antibody, the drug could not protect. The more likely explanation is that the treated individuals shed antiviral-resistant virus, so administration of drugs to the contacts was ineffective. Such a scenario was demonstrated to be the case years later[13] in a trial of rimantadine that was conducted over 2 years. In the treatment group, the index case was given drug, and the contacts were put on prophylaxis. In the control group, placebo was given to all family members. While there was a significant therapeutic effect in the index cases in the treatment group, with shortening of the duration of illness, no protective effect occurred in the contacts. Resistant virus was being shed by approximately 30% of those treated, and these resistant viruses spread to the contacts, rendering prophylaxis ineffective. Paradoxically, the therapeutic effect was present even when resistant virus was being shed. The resistant virus in the contact cases produced illness of expected virulence. Therefore, it can be concluded that these resistant viruses are 'fit' (ie, able to cause disease and transmit), but they are not more virulent than sensitive viruses.

Use of M2 Inhibitors in Closed Populations

Vaccine has a major effect in preventing serious consequences of influenza in frail, elderly residents. It also decreases the likelihood that an outbreak will occur. However, despite high levels of vaccination, outbreaks still occur in nursing homes, and, when they do take place, antivirals must be used to control them. Specific approaches to outbreak control are described in Chapter 14. Administration of rimantadine or amantadine to all residents with or without influenza-like illness has, in most circumstances, terminated the outbreak in several days. However, when the drugs are used in this way, some persons who are ill will shed resistant virus. The resistant virus will then transmit to individuals on prophylaxis, and prophylaxis will fail.[14] As a result, outbreaks will be prolonged; an example of this situation is shown in Figure 2. However, it is difficult to say how important the problem of viral resistance may be because the situation has changed with the availability of the neuraminidase inhibitors. As indicated in Chapter 14, if costs were not a consideration, the neuraminidase inhibitors would be the drugs of choice for treating those who are ill.

Resistance

The resistance frequently encountered with use of the M2 inhibitors is a result of amino acid substitutions in the transmembrane portion of the M2 protein.[15] Five positions where these substitutions can take place have been identified; some, such as the substitution of asparagine for serine at position 31, appear more often than others. At one time, the process of identifying resistant variants required identifying the viruses that were able to grow in the presence of the M2 inhibitor and sequencing them to identify the specific amino acid substitutions. Now it is possible to directly identify the substitutions, using the method of polymerase chain reaction followed by restriction analysis. It is accepted that these substitutions indicate that the virus is resistant.

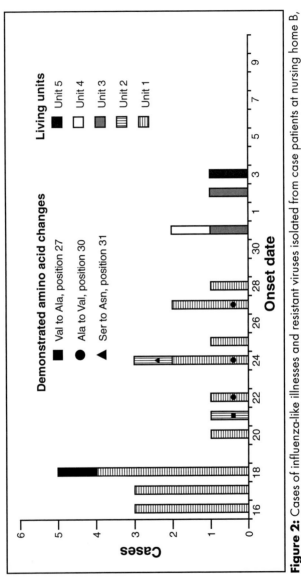

Figure 2: Cases of influenza-like illnesses and resistant viruses isolated from case patients at nursing home B, by living unit. Mast et al, *Am J Epidemiol* 1991;134:997.

Resistance is not produced when M2 inhibitors are used in prophylaxis. It has been estimated to occur in approximately 30% of patients on treatment, but the use of more sensitive techniques has demonstrated nearly universal occurrence of at least some level of resistance. Resistance to one M2 inhibitor will always be accompanied by resistance to the other. Although several lines of evidence suggested that the resistant viruses, while able to cause disease and transmit, might be at a competitive disadvantage to sensitive strains, this appeared to be a result of low volume of drug use. Recently increased frequency of resistance has been demonstrated, especially in Asia, of both seasonal viruses and A(H5N1) strains. These viruses mainly have a change at position 31.[16] Resistance also seems related to situations in which the virus is actively replicating, as in young children, who normally shed virus for long periods. Widespread use of M2 inhibitors, for example, in treatment during a pandemic, would lead to extensive transmission as well as production of resistant variants.

Side Effects

Most reports of adverse events related to the M2 inhibitors have come from prophylactic studies of healthy individuals. Fewer side effects have been seen in previously healthy adults treated for symptomatic influenza, in whom mild adverse events can be confused with the illness syndrome. Rimantadine is far less reactogenic than amantadine. In one study, withdrawals from 6 weeks of prophylaxis with rimantadine were similar to those from placebo, but, in another study, the percentage of withdrawals from rimantadine was 3.5%. Most side effects were related to the central nervous system (insomnia, impaired concentration, and nervousness); nausea and vomiting have also been reported. In a nursing home population given rimantadine for 6 weeks, it was difficult to see a difference from placebo until individual side effects were grouped.[3]

In contrast, amantadine has a higher frequency of side effects related to the central nervous system, estimated to be about 5% to 10%. The side effects appear to be not only more common, but also more severe. They have been a particular problem in nursing home patients, in whom 10.3% experienced confusion produced by amantadine vs 0.6% for rimantadine. The total percentage of adverse events was 18.6% and 1.9% for amantadine and rimantadine, respectively.[17]

Dosage

Amantadine and rimantadine are administered orally in prophylaxis and therapy at 200 mg daily in divided doses. In prophylaxis, both can be given once daily, as a result of their long half-lives, but the divided doses are thought to reduce the possibility of side effects. Divided doses are required in therapy, when rapid achievement of adequate blood levels is required. The recommended dosage of amantadine for children age 1 to 9 is up to 150 mg daily in a divided dose.

A reduction in dosage is recommended for both drugs when they are administered to the nursing home elderly; this applies to prophylaxis and therapy and assumes, for amantadine, a creatinine clearance greater than 50 mL/min/1.73 m². Dosages of amantadine for persons with reduced renal function are shown in Table 2. In persons on renal dialysis, the dosage should be 200 mg every 7 days; in nursing home elderly, reduction in dosage to 100 mg is advised.

With amantadine, the recommended dosage for prophylaxis in children aged 1 to 9 years is 2 to 4 mg/lb/day, without exceeding 150 mg/day. For children aged 9 to 12 years, the recommended dosage is 200 mg/day; however, many would support using the 100 mg/day dose in this age group.

Rimantadine is not approved for the treatment of children with influenza. The dosage for prophylaxis in those younger than 10 years is 5 mg/kg, without exceeding 150 mg daily, administered in a single dose. In children older than 10 years, the full adult dose can be given. Dosage should be reduced

Table 2: Dosage for Prophylaxis and Treatment of Uncomplicated Influenza A in Those With Impaired Renal Function

Creatinine Clearance (mL/min/1.73 m²)	Amantadine Dosage*
30-50	100 mg every day
15-29	100 mg every other day
<15	100 mg every 7 days

* After a 200-mg loading dose

to 100 mg/day in nursing home elderly, persons with severe hepatic dysfunction, and persons with renal failure (creatinine clearance ≤10 mL/min/1.73 m²). Therefore, reducing the dosage in persons with renal dysfunction is not as critical with rimantadine as with amantadine.

References

1. Monto AS, Gunn RA, Bandyk MG, et al: Prevention of Russian influenza by amantadine. *JAMA* 1979;241:1003-1007.

2. Dolin R, Reichman RC, Madore HP, et al: A controlled trial of amantadine and rimantadine in the prophylaxis of influenza A infection. *N Engl J Med* 1982;307:580-584.

3. Monto AS, Ohmit SE, Hornbuckle K, et al: Safety and efficacy of long-term use of rimantadine for prophylaxis of type A influenza in nursing homes. *Antimicrob Agents Chemother* 1995; 39:2224-2228.

4. Van Voris LP, Betts RF, Hayden FG, et al: Successful treatment of naturally occurring influenza A/USSR/77 H1N1. *JAMA* 1981; 245:1128-1131.

5. Hayden FG, Monto AS: Oral rimantadine hydrochloride therapy of influenza A virus H3N2 subtype infection in adults. *Antimicrob Agents Chemother* 1986;29:339-341.

6. Younkin SW, Betts RF, Roth FK, et al: Reduction in fever and symptoms in young adults with influenza A/Brazil/78 H1N1 infection after

treatment with aspirin or amantadine. *Antimicrob Agents Chemother* 1983;23:577-582.

7. Hayden FG, Hall WJ, Douglas RG Jr: Therapeutic effects of aerosolized amantadine in naturally acquired infection due to influenza A virus. *J Infect Dis* 1980;141:535-542.

8. Thompson J, Fleet L, Lawrence E, et al: A comparison of acetaminophen and rimantadine in the treatment of influenza A infection in children. *J Med Virol* 1987;21:249-255.

9. Hall CB, Dolin R, Gala CL, et al: Children with influenza A infection: treatment with rimantadine. *Pediatrics* 1987;80:275-282.

10. Hayden FG, Sperber SJ, Belshe RB, et al: Recovery of drug-resistant influenza A virus during therapeutic use of rimantadine. *Antimicrob Agents Chemother* 1991;35:1741-1747.

11. Galbraith AW, Oxford JS, Schild GC, et al: Protective effect of 1-adamantanamine hydrochloride on influenza A2 infections in the family environment: a controlled double-blind study. *Lancet* 1969;2:1026-1028.

12. Galbraith AW, Oxford JS, Schild GC, et al: Study of 1-adamantanamine hydrochloride used prophylactically during the Hong Kong influenza epidemic in the family environment. *Bull World Health Organ* 1969;41:677-682.

13. Hayden FG, Belshe RB, Clover RD, et al: Emergence and apparent transmission of rimantadine-resistant influenza A virus in families. *N Engl J Med* 1989;321:1696-1702.

14. Mast EE, Harmon MW, Gravenstein S, et al: Emergence and possible transmission of amantadine-resistant viruses during nursing home outbreaks of influenza A (H3N2). *Am J Epidemiol* 1991;134:988-997.

15. Hay AJ, Zambon MC, Wolstenholme AJ, et al: Molecular basis of resistance of influenza A viruses to amantadine. *J Antimicrob Chemother* 1986;18:19-29.

16. Bright RA, Medina MJ, Xu X, et al: Incidence of amantadine resistance among influenza A(H3N2) viruses isolated worldwide from 1994 to 2005: a cause for concern. *Lancet* 2005;366:1175-1181.

17. Keyser LA, Karl M, Nafziger AN, et al: Comparison of central nervous system adverse effects of amantadine and rimantadine used as sequential prophylaxis of influenza A in elderly nursing home patients. *Arch Intern Med* 2000;160:1485-1488.

Chapter 13

Neuraminidase Inhibitors

The M2 inhibitors, amantadine (Symmetrel®) and rimantadine (Flumadine®), are effective in prophylaxis and therapy of type A influenza. However, they have a number of limitations, in addition to their restriction to type A influenza. As indicated in the previous chapter, their precise efficacy in treatment is difficult to quantify because of the way they were studied. They have not been demonstrated to prevent complications, and they have some degree of reactogenicity, which can be a problem with amantadine. Additionally, treatment with the M2 inhibitors predictably produces resistance, and the resistant virus, while no more virulent than the sensitive strains, can be transmitted. Therefore, the new class of antivirals, the neuraminidase inhibitors (NAIs), is considered an important advance, especially in the therapy of influenza.

Efficacy of NAIs in Prophylaxis

Seasonal use is the most efficient method of determining the efficacy of an influenza antiviral in prophylaxis. As discussed with the M2 inhibitors, it is not likely that the drug will be used for periods of a month or longer, except in certain situations, but its use throughout an outbreak gives the best estimate of its value in disease prevention. Studies of zanamivir (Relenza®) and oseltamivir (Tamiflu®) were designed using prior studies of the M2 inhibitors as models. Zanamivir was evaluated at two sites, the University of

13

Table 1: Efficacy of Seasonal Prophylaxis of Influenza With Zanamivir (4 weeks) and Oseltamivir (6 weeks)

	Zanamivir	Oseltamivir
Prevention of symptomatic laboratory-confirmed influenza	67%	74%
Prevention of influenza with fever	84%	82%

Lin et al, *Arch Intern Med* 2001;161:441-446; Fine et al, *Clin Infect Dis* 2001;32:1784-1791.

Michigan and the University of Missouri, over a period of 4 weeks.[1] The primary end point was termed *laboratory-confirmed clinical influenza* and did not require fever; a secondary end point that required fever was also determined. Laboratory confirmation meant either virus isolation or a fourfold rise in antibody titer. Results for both end points are shown in Table 1. The preventive efficacy of zanamivir for confirmed influenza illness was 67%; when the analysis was restricted to more severe illnesses with fever, preventive efficacy rose to 84%.

The seasonal trials of oseltamivir were conducted in several centers based in Virginia and Texas.[2] In one area, there was a major outbreak, while in the other, there was little illness. The data were analyzed separately and together. The end points used required more symptoms than those used in the zanamivir study. Overall, 74% of laboratory-confirmed illnesses were prevented by oseltamivir (Table 1). When fever was required as in the zanamivir study, the rate rose to 82%. Because of the variation in the attack rates at the two sites, the protective efficacy shown in Virginia was higher than that shown in the table (82% for all laboratory-confirmed disease without fever). Also not shown in the table is the effect of the drugs on total infection rates (ie, symptomatic and asymptomatic infections). As with the M2 inhibitors, asymptomatic infections that produce protective antibodies occur. Total infections were reduced by 31% with zanamivir and by 50% with oseltamivir. Thus, it can be concluded that the NAIs are roughly equivalent to each other in prophylaxis. They are also similar in this regard to the M2 inhibitors; however, they protect against type B influenza viruses, which the M2 inhibitors do not.

Household Prophylaxis

A more practical approach to use of these antivirals in prophylaxis would be over a shorter time, during the peak of an outbreak. Members of a family in which a case of influenza has occurred are at increased risk of illness. Most disease transmission will be intrafamilial, but some cases will be newly introduced. In either situation, prophylaxis can be used in the household for a limited period, typically 10 days, to successfully prevent transmission. In the first such evaluation of zanamivir, the first case in the household, or the index case, was placed on zanamivir for treatment, and the rest of the household members aged 5 years or older were placed on placebo. This method allows assessment of the effect on the treated case as well as prophylactic efficacy in the contacts. The efficacy in preventing influenza illnesses varied from 72% to 87% according to the end point used. All of these results were statistically significant. For the intent-to-treat population, efficacy was 79%.[3]

With oseltamivir, the first study design was different.[4] The contacts were given prophylaxis, and the index case was not treated. Protective efficacy ranged between 84% and 89%, again depending on the end point. More recently, zanamivir was tested in households without treating the index case, and a trial of oseltamivir was conducted in which the index case was always treated but the contacts were randomized to prophylaxis or placebo. In each case, results were similar to those seen in previous studies, indicating that reduction of virus shedding in the index case is not a major factor in the observed reduction of infection in the contacts, who will need prophylaxis in order to be protected. In no case was resistance a problem in these trials. Short-term, targeted prophylaxis in which prophylaxis is given to the contacts is an attractive option for use not only in the family, but also, possibly, in similar settings, including the workplace.

Use of the NAIs in Therapy

Evaluation of the NAIs' value in therapy was conducted on a far larger scale than that of the M2 inhibitors and followed the now-standard study design for new drugs. Phase II studies of zanamivir were intended not only to determine efficacy, but also to identify whether a combined intranasal-inhaled dose was superior to an inhaled dose.[5] There was no advantage detected in the combined approach, so further study involved only a twice-daily dose of 10 mg of zanamivir as the standard treatment dose. No such issues affected oseltamivir, which is administered orally. For oseltamivir, the only question to be settled was one of finding the proper dose. Early studies determined that there was little advantage to increasing the dose beyond 75 mg b.i.d.

Efficacy of both drugs was evaluated, by agreement with the US Food and Drug Administration (FDA), with an end point termed 'alleviation of symptoms.' The detailed specifics of the alleviation end point differed between zanamivir and oseltamivir; for example, lack of fever was included in the definition for zanamivir but not in that for oseltamivir. Also, with zanamivir, the drug was used within 48 hours of illness onset, while with oseltamivir, recruitment into trials was carried out within 36 hours. An illustration of the concept of the alleviation end points is shown in Table 2. However, despite differences in the drugs' mode of administration, pharmacokinetics, and possible side effects, the results of the treatment studies were remarkably similar.

Table 2: Alleviation End Point

- Creates a single artificial point for each patient
- Slightly different for zanamivir and oseltamivir
  - Zanamivir: no fever; mild or no cough, sore throat, headache, or myalgia
  - Oseltamivir: mild or no cough, nasal obstruction, sore throat, fatigue, headache, myalgia, or feverishness
- Status maintained for 24 hours
- Independent of any 'relief medications' taken
- Medians calculated for groups—days for zanamivir, hours for oseltamivir

Shortening of Illness Duration

Zanamivir treatment was evaluated in three efficacy studies. There were minor differences in design, such as some sites requiring that participants have reports of feverishness rather than documented fever. All three studies were conducted in mainly healthy adults, with few exclusions, so that small numbers of individuals with risk conditions were included. All identified a shortening of illness duration of approximately 1 to 1.5 days to the point of alleviation. One of the largest studies was conducted mainly in North America. Although the point estimates of the reduction in duration were similar to those in other studies, there was a great deal of variability in the data, which resulted in the differences between groups in this particular study not being statistically significant. Various explanations for these results have been offered, including laboratory data. For example, if cases identified as positive by the polymerase chain reaction technique were excluded, the results became significant. Taken together, however, all three studies showed a clear advantage to treatment.

In fact, a European-based study not only was statistically significant, but also identified a reduction in illness duration of 2.5 days.[6]

To answer any questions concerning efficacy, and to take advantage of a large data set to identify special groups who would benefit from drug treatment, a pooled analysis of all Phase II and III studies was carried out.[7] Pooled analyses are different in methodology from meta-analyses, in that data from individuals are used instead of grouped data from each study being combined. Pooled analysis is considered a more powerful technique and is used if individual data are available. The reduction in illness duration in the overall population of those with laboratory-confirmed influenza illness was 1 day. However, subset analysis of this group showed that differences were greater for persons with fever, in whom the reduction was 1.5 days, and for persons considered severely ill at outset, in whom the reduction was 3 days.

Relief medications were made available to both treatment and placebo groups in the efficacy studies, and their use was originally not considered in determining when alleviation occurred. In fact, taking relief medications has been used as an end point in these analyses, with those on antivirals using less antipyretic and cough medication than those on placebo. The alleviation end point in the zanamivir study was reanalyzed, with the added requirement that relief medications not be used.[8] Results are shown in Figure 1. The reduction in duration was 2 days for all influenza-positive participants. However, in some subsets of this group, reduction in duration was much greater. This greater effect was a result of illness duration being longer in untreated participants in each of these subsets; that is, there was a greater ability to shorten duration because, without treatment, the illness would have been longer. Higher-risk individuals, older persons, and persons with underlying conditions were not recruitment targets, but small numbers of these individuals were included in the

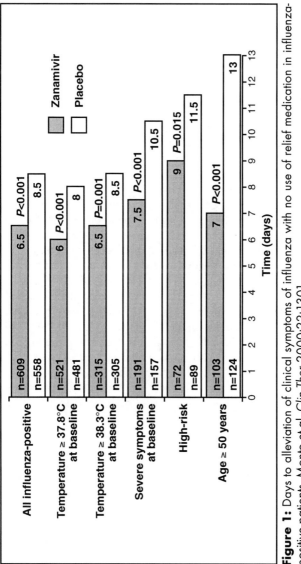

Figure 1: Days to alleviation of clinical symptoms of influenza with no use of relief medication in influenza-positive patients. Monto et al, *Clin Ther* 2000;22:1301.

studies. There was a reduction in illness duration of 2.5 to 5 days in this group.

Alleviation, as defined for study purposes, does not occur until influenza illness has been present for many days. The question is whether symptoms are reduced before alleviation. Figure 2 shows that after 1 day of therapy, there were already statistically significant differences in symptom scores. These differences increase over time. It is because of these differences that relief medications were used less in those treated with NAIs.

Oseltamivir in Therapy

Prelicensure studies of oseltamivir were conducted over a much shorter period of time but also involved large numbers of participants. Two studies, one in the United States and the other in rest of the world, used the same alleviation end point but also examined other outcomes.[9,10] In the US study, as shown in Table 3, duration of illness to alleviation was reduced by 1.3 days in patients given the approved dose of 75 mg b.i.d. Time to return to normal activities was reduced by almost 3 days. There was also a reduction in duration of illness of 1.3 days in the study conducted in the rest of the world, with similar reduction in time to become afebrile and return to normal sleep patterns. Each of these studies, for the first time, suggested that oseltamivir prevents complications of influenza, especially those requiring antibiotics. These findings add to the value of using NAIs to treat influenza.

Pediatric Studies

Influenza morbidity is highest in children, and pediatric illness is often of longer duration, with prolonged viral shedding. Studies of zanamivir in children have been age limited because drug administration requires use of an inhaler device.[11] The studies were carried out in children as young as 5 years, but approval for pediatric use in the United States is only for children aged 7 years and older.

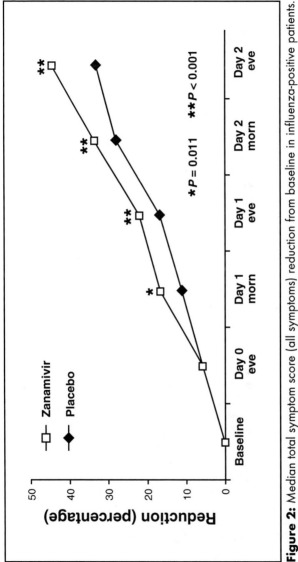

Figure 2: Median total symptom score (all symptoms) reduction from baseline in influenza-positive patients. (GlaxoSmithKline personal communication.)

Table 3: Duration in Hours (Days) and Severity of Influenza in Placebo- and Oseltamivir- Treated Infected Patients in a US Study

	Placebo n = 129
Median duration of illness	103 (4.3)
Median time to return to normal activity	225 (9.4)

Adapted from Treanor et al, *JAMA* 2000;283:1016-1024.

Results of the pediatric studies mirrored those of the adult studies. Contrary to expectations, no greater reduction in duration of illness was demonstrated.

A liquid formulation of oseltamivir was evaluated in children as young as 1 year. In this study, end points might have been more difficult to determine because they relied on physician observation rather than patients' reports of symptoms.[12] As can be seen in Table 4, the reduction in duration of influenza to alleviation was 1.5 days, not much different from that observed in adults. However, there were critical findings concerning prevention of one of the most frequent conditions of young children, acute otitis media. Overall occurrence of otitis media was reduced by 44%, and otitis media confirmed by tympanometry was reduced by 50%. There was also a 40% reduction in antibiotic treatment for all physician-diagnosed complications. It should be remembered that these decreases were observed in children being treated for influenza, not in primary pre-

Oseltamivir 75 mg b.i.d. n = 124	Oseltamivir 150 mg b.i.d. n = 121
72* (3.0)	70* (2.9)
157** (6.5)	180** (7.5)

* $P <0.01$
** $P <0.05$

vention. The results offer hope for preventing important complications of influenza in children and reducing use of antibiotics.

Other Population Groups

Large studies have not been conducted in other groups, but there have been smaller studies or observations of effects of both NAIs since licensure. Of greatest interest are the groups at higher risk of complications, the usual recipients of influenza vaccine. Reports of bronchospasm with zanamivir have resulted in warnings from the FDA. A study of zanamivir in asthma patients has therefore been of particular importance. This study, conducted mainly in adult asthma patients and some individuals with chronic obstructive pulmonary disease, showed a time to alleviation of 1.5 days.[13] The drug also resulted in one less night of sleep disturbance. No evidence of exacerbation of asthma was seen in 215 individuals with diagnosed asthma who

13

received zanamivir. While encouraging, these results do not help resolve the issue of bronchospasm because the reports to the FDA have been infrequent, and the number of patients in the study was small.

Data on other high-risk individuals, including older individuals, are more limited. High-risk status was generally not an exclusion from the Phase II and III clinical trials of zanamivir, so it is possible to examine data from those individuals for indications of differences in symptom resolution. As mentioned above, because of longer duration of illness in such populations, there was greater alleviation of symptoms. Also, when evaluated in terms of rapidity of symptom resolution, clear differences were seen in those with risk conditions and in persons ≥ 50 years of age.

Prevention of Complications by NAI Treatment

Influenza is a major health problem not only for the primary illness it produces, but also because its complications sometimes lead to hospitalization and death. Symptomatic therapy may reduce some manifestations of illness, and the M2 inhibitors do have clear effects in shortening the duration of type A influenza. However, the M2 inhibitors have not been shown to affect complications, especially those requiring antibiotics. As indicated above, oseltamivir has been shown to have a major effect in preventing otitis media in children with influenza; no such observations have been made with zanamivir in children. This is partly because the zanamivir trials were restricted to children 5 years or older, a result of the fact that the drug is delivered by oral inhalation. However, zanamivir and oseltamivir have each been shown to prevent lower respiratory complications. The reduction in complications leading to antibiotic usage was examined in a pooled analysis of participation in the zanamivir treatment studies.[14] Upper respiratory events were reduced by only 10%; there was no reduction in sinusitis. However, there was a 40% reduction in lower respiratory complications, a combination of acute bronchitis and pneumonia.

Table 4: Reduction in Events Following Oseltamivir Treatment of Children 1 to 12 Years of Age

End Point	Reductions
Illness duration until alleviation	1.5 days
Duration of fever	1.1 days
Physician-diagnosed complications requiring antibiotics	40%
Physician-diagnosed otitis media	44%
Tympanometry-confirmed otitis media	50%

Miller et al, *Clin Infect Dis* 2000;31:433-438.

Secondary complications were reduced by oseltamivir in all age groups, with a reduction of 40% in children, 51% in adults, and 20% in smaller numbers of older adults. Data on reduction of complications in adults shown in Table 5. There are also emerging indications that oseltamivir may prevent hospitalizations, which would be expected because hospitalizations usually result from pneumonia.

NAIs in Nursing Home Populations

Oseltamivir has been studied for seasonal prophylaxis in the frail elderly (ie, nursing home residents). The intent was to demonstrate that the drug protected vaccinated individuals against influenza over a 6-week period. This represents seasonal prophylaxis in a nursing home and is only possible because vaccine in this population does not completely protect against influenza illness. The efficacy of the drug in this setting was 91%, and there was good tolerability in the 276 individuals receiving the drug.

Seasonal prophylaxis is an excellent way of preventing an influenza outbreak in a frail nursing home population.

Table 5: Efficacy of Oseltamivir in Preventing Lower Respiratory Tract Complications (LRTCs) Leading to Antibiotic Use

	Percent Reduction		
LRTCs Leading to Antibiotic Use	Overall n=2,413	Otherwise Healthy n=1,644	At Risk n=769
All LRTC	**55%***	**67 %***	**34%†**
Bronchitis	52%	60%	34%
Pneumonia	61%	77%	30%
Influenza A	**55%**	**63%**	**34%**
Influenza B	**54%**	**71%**	**25%**

* Comparison of oseltamivir vs placebo, P<.001.

† Comparison of oseltamivir vs placebo, P=.02.

Kaiser L, et al. Arch Intern Med. 2003; 163:1667-72.

However, the most common use of antivirals in this population will be outbreak control, in which drug use will be initiated for a limited period after virus transmission in the facility has been recognized. There have been many reports of using the M2 inhibitors for this purpose. Oseltamivir has been successfully employed in outbreak control in US nursing homes involving a total of almost 1,000 individuals. The approach is similar to that used for the M2 inhibitors. After the outbreak is recognized by rapid tests and, ideally, confirmed by standard laboratory tests, those with illness are given 75 mg of the drug twice daily, and the rest of the residents are given a prophylactic dose of 75 mg daily. The treatment is maintained for 5 days and the prophylaxis for 15 days. This strategy may need adaptation as more experience is gained.

Zanamivir has been compared with rimantadine in nursing home outbreak control. Consenting individuals were randomized to one of these two drugs. The remaining residents were given the M2 inhibitor. Zanamivir appeared more efficacious in this setting, mainly because of emergence of resistance to the M2 inhibitor, which rendered that drug ineffective. Thus, the NAIs both appear to be ideal choices for outbreak control in a setting where M2 resistance may develop. For zanamivir, the ability of this population to use the inhalation device may be a consideration.

Resistance to the NAIs

Resistance to both zanamivir and oseltamivir can be produced easily in the test tube, but it has not been seen frequently in studies in humans or laboratory animals. A zanamivir-resistant type B virus was isolated from an immunosuppressed child who had chronic shedding of the virus.[15] There were mutations found in the hemagglutinin and neuraminidase of this virus. So far, no other strain resistant to zanamivir has been isolated. There is a debate concerning whether this is a result of resistance being an unusually infrequent occurrence or of the fact that attempts to identify resistant virus on day 5 of treatment have been limited. There is truth in both views, but it is as yet impossible to say which is more correct.

Oseltamivir resistance has been demonstrated more frequently; studies have routinely involved attempts to isolate resistant viruses late in treatment. Children have a longer course of infection, and in a pediatric study, 3% to 5% of viruses were resistant. Resistance has been seen in type A(H3N2) and type A(H1N1) viruses and is associated with amino acid substitutions in the viral neuraminidase.[16]

In another pediatric study, conducted in Japan with a reduced dose of oseltamivir, 16% of children shed resistant A(H1N1) virus. However, resistant viruses appear often to not be 'fit,' which means that they have lower infectability and ability to transmit than the sensitive strains.

Further attention must be paid to use of zanamivir and oseltamivir in the immunosuppressed. It is likely that if resistance is to occur, it will be detected in this population. The major question concerning resistance is whether, with increasing antiviral use, it will become more and more common. To make sure this is not occurring, a network has been established to follow a large sample of viruses from around the world. Although funded by manufacturers, it is independent and includes representatives from the World Health Organization and its Collaborating Centers.[17]

Side Effects of the NAIs

Zanamivir is only partially absorbed following inhalation. Side effects have been infrequent in clinical trials; in many studies, there was no difference between the treated group and those on placebo. However, since licensure, there have been rare reports of bronchospasm, mainly in persons with underlying bronchial hyperactivity, but also in some individuals without such conditions. Because these are spontaneous reports, and because the individuals were already infected with influenza, it is hard to quantify the occurrence of these events and to determine their causal relationship to the drug. No study of reasonable size would be able to unravel the relationship because the frequency of bronchospasm is so low. It is also not clear whether, if there is a relationship, it is with the drug or the lactose carrier. The current recommendation for patients with asthma who use inhaled medications is that they use their respiratory inhaler before they take zanamivir.

Oseltamivir is bioavailable, and the carboxylate is widely distributed. The most commonly reported side effect is one of nausea, sometimes accompanied by vomiting. Frequencies have varied greatly depending on the population and study design; unlike the situation with the M2 inhibitors, treatment studies have reported the same or higher rates of gastrointestinal side effects as the prophylactic studies. Gastrointestinal side effects have generally been graded mild to moderate and mostly occur in the first 2 days of administration. Eating a snack with the dose is effective in lowering the frequency of nausea. This may account for the variability in reporting gastrointestinal symptoms. Even when they occur (4% for nausea without vomiting and 6% for vomiting), there has been less than 1% excess withdrawal from the clinical trials by those on drug. In other respects, the drug is well tolerated, with little or no difference between those on drug and those on placebo. Drug-drug interactions have not been reported.

Dosage and Administration

Zanamivir is given by inhalation using a Diskhaler® device. A Rotadisk® containing blisters with medication is loaded into the device. One blister is punctured by the device, and the patient breathes in vigorously to inhale the medication. Each blister contains 5 mg of the active ingredient. Each dosing episode consists of two inhalations. The Diskhaler® rotates the disk after each inhalation. The drug is approved for treatment only within 2 days of illness onset and can be used at the regular dose of 10 mg (two inhalations) twice daily for 5 days. There is no dose reduction in children; it is approved down to age 7 years. On the first day of therapy, the full two doses should be given, as long as they are 2 hours apart.

Oseltamivir is licensed for therapy and prophylaxis. For treatment, it is approved down to age 1 year within 2 days of onset of illness. For prophylaxis, it is approved for patients 13 years and older. Dosage in prophylaxis is 75 mg daily for at least 7 days; it can be used for up to 6 weeks. In therapy, 75 mg twice daily should be given to those 13 years and older. Dosage in children is calculated based on weight and may require use of an oral suspension. The full dose may be given to patients who weigh more than 40 kg (88 lb). A lower dose schedule is provided with the pediatric suspension.

Since the drug is mostly excreted renally, dose reduction may be necessary for those with decreased kidney function. No reduction is necessary for those with creatinine clearance above 30 mL/min/1.73 m^2. For those with creatinine clearance between 10 and 30 mL/min/1.73 m^2, the therapy dose should be reduced to 75 mg once daily and the prophylaxis dose should be reduced to 75 mg every other day. There are no recommendations for those with end-stage renal disease or on routine hemodialysis.

References

1. Monto AS, Robinson DP, Herlocher ML, et al: Zanamivir in the prevention of influenza among healthy adults: a randomized controlled trial. *JAMA* 1999;282:31-35.

2. Hayden FG, Atmar RL, Schilling M, et al: Use of the selective oral neuraminidase inhibitor oseltamivir to prevent influenza. *N Engl J Med* 1999;341:1336-1343.

3. Hayden FG, Gubareva LV, Monto AS, et al: Inhaled zanamivir for the prevention of influenza in families. Zanamivir Family Study Group. *N Engl J Med* 2000;343:1282-1289.

4. Wellivir R, Monto AS, Carewicz O, et al: Effectiveness of oseltamivir in preventing influenza in household contacts: a randomized controlled trial. *JAMA* 2001;285:748-754.

5. Monto AS, Fleming DM, Henry D, et al: Efficacy and safety of the neuraminidase inhibitor zanamivir in the treatment of influenza A and B virus infections. *J Infect Dis* 1999;180:254-261.

6. Mäkelä MJ, Pauksens K, Rostila T, et al: Clinical efficacy and safety of the orally inhaled neuraminidase inhibitor zanamivir in the treatment of influenza: a randomized, double-blind, placebo-controlled European study. *J Infect* 2000;40:42-48.

7. Monto AS, Webster A, Keene O: Randomized, placebo-controlled studies of inhaled zanamivir in the treatment of influenza A and B: pooled efficacy analysis. *J Antimicrob Chemother* 1999;44: 23-29.

8. Monto AS, Moult AB, Sharp SJ: Effect of zanamivir on duration and resolution of influenza symptoms. *Clin Ther* 2000;22:1294-1305.

9. Treanor JJ, Hayden FG, Vrooman PS, et al: Efficacy and safety of the oral neuraminidase inhibitor oseltamivir in treating acute influenza: a randomized controlled trial. US Oral Neuraminidase Study Group. *JAMA* 2000;283:1016-1024.

10. Nicholson KG, Aoki FY, Osterhaus AD, et al: Efficacy and safety of oseltamivir in treatment of acute influenza: a randomised controlled trial. Neuraminidase Inhibitor Flu Treatment Investigator Group. *Lancet* 2000;355:1845-1850.

11. Hedrick JA, Barzilai A, Behre U, et al: Zanamivir for treatment of symptomatic influenza A and B infection in children five to twelve years of age: a randomized controlled trial. *Pediatr Infect Dis J* 2000;19:410-417.

12. Whitley RJ, Hayden FG, Reisinger KS, et al: Oral oseltamivir treatment of influenza in children. *Pediatr Infect Dis J* 2001;20:127-133.

13. Murphy KR, Eivindson A, Pauksens K, et al: Efficacy and safety of inhaled zanamivir for the treatment of influenza in patients with asthma or chronic obstructive pulmonary disease. *Clin Drug Invest* 2000;20:337-349.

14. Kaiser L, Keene ON, Hammond JM, et al: Impact of zanamivir on antibiotic use for respiratory events following acute influenza in adolescents and adults. *Arch Intern Med* 2000;160:3234-3240.

15. Gubareva LV, Matrosovich MN, Brenner MK, et al: Evidence for zanamivir resistance in an immunocompromised child infected with influenza B virus. *J Infect Dis* 1998;178:1257-1262.

16. Gubareva LV, Kaiser L, Matrosovich MN, et al: Selection of influenza virus mutants in experimentally infected volunteers treated with oseltamivir. *J Infect Dis* 2001;183:523-531.

17. Zambon M, Hayden FG: Position statement: global neuraminidase inhibitor susceptibility network. *Antiviral Res* 2001;49:147-156.

13

Chapter **14**

Special Populations

Groups at Risk of Complications

Influenza has particularly severe effects on certain groups in terms of morbidity and mortality. These groups have been discussed in the epidemiology and vaccination chapters. Of particular importance are those who are at higher risk of developing complications from influenza infection, including older individuals and those who have chronic cardiovascular system disease. These individuals should be vaccinated each year. However, the inactivated vaccine is about 70% to 90% efficacious. Therefore, there will be cases of influenza among the vaccinated as well as the unvaccinated. Disease occurring in high-risk, vaccinated individuals was sometimes treated with the M2 inhibitors. Now that the neuraminidase inhibitors (NAIs) have been demonstrated to prevent complications, it seems most appropriate to use them to treat high-risk patients as a regular practice. While the prevention of complications may not be as dramatic as in healthy individuals, patients with risk conditions have been shown to have a greater shortening of illness duration because the illness lasts longer in such persons, and, therefore, drugs can have a more dramatic effect when they shorten it. In older individuals and those with underlying illnesses, a serious infection like influenza can have serious long-term effects; any significant reduction in severity of such an illness can prevent deterioration.

Immunosuppression

Differences in the severity and chronicity of influenza in immunosuppressed patients will vary based on the degree and characteristics of immunosuppression. Human immunodeficiency virus (HIV) infection is one of the most common forms of acquired immunosuppression in many parts of the world. In theory, defects in cell-mediated immunity associated with HIV infection should have a major effect on the course of influenza, given the role of such immunity in recovery. It is therefore surprising that there have been conflicting data on whether those with HIV experience more severe illness when infected with influenza. A possible explanation for these conflicts may be associated with the stage of HIV infection. One study suggested that mortality in those with HIV infection goes up significantly in the influenza season and that death certificate diagnoses were compatible with influenza.[1] Other studies directly following individuals with HIV have indicated that this group does not suffer more profound illness than individuals who are not HIV infected.[2] Still others report the serious effects of influenza in a series of individuals with HIV infection. The conclusion is that those with HIV infection should be vaccinated because no harm and perhaps major benefit will result. As long as clinical acquired immunodeficiency syndrome has not developed, antibody response will be unaffected. However, when CD4 counts drop below 100 or HIV RNA copies rise above 100,000 per mL, response is unlikely. Prophylaxis with an antiviral should be considered in this situation.[3]

Influenza is nearly always a self-limited infection; even when late complications develop, it is rare that chronic viral infection is responsible. One exception occurs in those with bone marrow or solid organ transplants or hematologic malignancy. Use of steroid boluses and other forms of immunosuppression is associated with these situations.[4] Fatal pneumonias in these cases are viral in etiology, not bacte-

14

rial. Many of these influenza infections are nosocomial, again reinforcing the need for vaccination of health-care workers. Long-term shedding of virus in immunocompromised individuals needs to be treated; chronic shedding has been reported to last for up to 5 months. Success in ending the infection has been reported occasionally, but until the NAIs were developed, the difficulty often encountered was development of resistance to the M2 inhibitors.[5] This could be expected, given that under ordinary circumstances, at least 30% of those treated with the M2 inhibitors develop resistant illness, and resistance in circulatory type A viruses has increased.

Resistance is much less common with the NAIs, which can be used to treat type B infection as well as type A. However, resistance to the NAIs may develop. There has been one report of a child with chronic type B influenza infection treated with zanamivir (Relenza®). The patient, an 18-month-old girl, developed the influenza infection following bone marrow transplantation. She was treated with nebulized zanamivir for 2 weeks but continued to shed virus. The type B virus had changes in both neuraminidase and hemagglutinin, which indicates that resistance may be a problem in this type of patient.[6] Oseltamivir (Tamiflu®) is more likely to be used in this situation because of the way it is delivered. One way to delay development of antiviral resistance in type A viruses would be to use an NAI and an M2 inhibitor together.

Influenza in Nursing Homes

Nursing homes place individuals with increased susceptibility to influenza in a setting where transmission is facilitated by residents' proximity to each other and close contact with staff members. Vaccination is strongly recommended for residents and for staff. In recent years, residents' vaccination rates have steadily increased, largely as a result of Medicare coverage and the decision to not require informed consent of residents or their surrogate decision makers. Most homes have developed a system for offering vaccine in mid-autumn. The most successful homes also offer vaccine to newly admitted residents until there is local influenza activity. In the past, the recommendation has been to delay vaccination until late October or early November because of evidence that vaccination given closer to an outbreak increases the likelihood of protection.[7] In recent years, careful scheduling of vaccination has been impossible because of vaccine shortages and delays. Later vaccination is probably better for the resident, but it is better to be vaccinated early than not at all. Revaccination of an individual during a late influenza season will not result in increased protection. One inoculation per season is sufficient.[8]

As indicated in Chapter 9, influenza outbreaks still occur in nursing homes with high vaccination rates, despite the fact that vaccination of most of the residents should augment the protection produced by individual vaccination. The reason outbreaks still occur, particularly with A(H3N2) viruses, must have something to do with the virulence of these particular viruses. However, the main factor is the frail status of the residents and what has loosely been termed *immune senescence*.[9] Vaccination of staff is therefore necessary because the staff introduce infection into the home from the outside. One study has shown that health worker vaccination is more important than resident vaccination.[10] However, vaccination of staff has been difficult to accomplish in the United States, especially because of high staff turnover. In Canada, vaccination can be made a condition of employment, but this approach is harder to implement in the United States. Therefore, incentives must be found to increase staff vaccination. Financial incentives may even be cost-effective when compared to the cost of an outbreak. However, high resident vaccination rates should be maintained. Vaccination may not prevent uncomplicated influenza very well in nursing home residents, but it does protect against complications, such as pneumonia, and against death.[11]

14

Table 1: Calendar of Events in Nursing Homes

September-November
- Institute vaccine program for residents and staff.
- Continue vaccination program until influenza terminates in community.

October-April
- Maintain surveillance of influenza in home.

November
- Hold in-service training for staff on steps for recognition and control of outbreaks.
- Write standing orders for use of antivirals.

An outbreak of influenza in a nursing home is an emergency and requires immediate action. However, outbreak control receives less attention than vaccination programs in many nursing homes. All nursing homes should have plans in place for combating outbreaks. A rough guide to the essential elements of outbreak control is shown in Table 1. Because staff turnover is so rapid, it is critical to have annual in-service staff training to review the essentials of illness recognition, the availability of diagnostic tests, and the components of outbreak control. Standing orders for the use of antivirals in a declared outbreak should be written. In addition, the kidney function of each resident should be assessed because amantadine (Symmetrel®) and, to a lesser extent, oseltamivir must be given at reduced dosage in patients with renal insufficiency. In current approaches to control, it should be remembered that the adamantanes are of extremely limited utility because most type A viruses are now resistant to this class of drugs.

Surveillance should begin according to the calendar, not following recognition of community outbreaks. Often, community outbreaks are first recognized in a nursing home. Fever and cough are the hallmarks of influenza in younger groups; however, it is common for fever not to be observed in nursing home residents with documented influenza illness. One system of recognizing influenza that has been applied with success is collection of specimens for viral identification from residents with cough and a fever of 99.5°F and residents who have onset of cough. Clinical judgment, of course, is required to assess other indicators of change in overall status, often an early indicator of influenza. While the rapid antigen detection tests are not ideally sensitive and can be nonspecific, they appear to offer balancing advantages in the nursing home setting, where speed is necessary. There needs to be an evaluation of tests that are waived under the Clinical Laboratory Improvement Act in the nursing home setting because, according to legal regulations, other tests cannot be performed there.

The number of identified cases of influenza recommended to declare an outbreak varies. A cluster of two or more positive rapid tests in a small home or on a separate wing of a large home should be sufficient to declare that transmission is occurring, given these tests' known lower sensitivity in older individuals. Whenever possible, specimens should be sent to a virus laboratory to confirm that influenza is present and to type the virus as A or B, which some of the rapid tests do not do. This would be critical if the antiviral to be used for outbreak control is an M2 inhibitor, especially since increased resistance in circulatory viruses has been documented.

14

The declaration of an influenza outbreak in a nursing home should result in the immediate implementation of various activities. It is often stated that vaccine should be offered again. However, a continuing vaccination program that made vaccine available before the outbreak would have the advantage of reducing the likelihood of an outbreak in the first place. Environmental measures should be put into place. These include isolation or cohorting of cases

Table 2: Antivirals for Outbreak Control

Drug	Dose (prophylaxis)	Observations
M2 Inhibitors[†]		
Amantadine (Symmetrel®)	100 mg daily	Use with caution in renal insufficiency; may cause central nervous system side effects
Rimantadine (Flumadine®)	100 mg daily	Rare convulsions
Neuraminidase Inhibitors		
Zanamivir (Relenza®)	10 mg daily (not yet approved in United States for this use)	Patient must be able to inhale deeply (two inhalations)
Oseltamivir (Tamiflu®)	75 mg daily	Give with food; use with caution in marked renal insufficiency

[†]Use of drugs limited by resistance

and institution of droplet precautions. Admissions to the facility should be stopped during this period.

While helpful, none of these measures by themselves will terminate an established outbreak. Termination requires the use of antivirals, which have a mechanism of action that is totally different from that of vaccine. It has been shown repeatedly that the effect of antivirals in prophylaxis is at least additive to the effect of vaccine, even when there is a good match between the virus in the vaccine and that in circulation. Therefore, antivirals should be given to everyone in the facility or the affected unit, regardless of vaccination status. Most residents will be uninfected, some will be ill, and some will be in the incubation period. Any antiviral can be used in a type A outbreak; only the NAIs can be used in a type B outbreak. A list of the available drugs and their cautions is shown in Table 2.

Resistance to the M2 inhibitors has occurred in nursing homes, sometimes leading to failure of prophylaxis. The NAIs would therefore be preferred, except for their higher price. Unfortunately, costs are a major consideration in nursing homes. Thus, the M2 inhibitors may still be employed, but they must be used with caution. The cheapest, amantadine, can produce central nervous system side effects, even when the reduced dose of 100 mg is used and careful attention is paid to renal function (see Chapter 12). These side effects can lead to falls in mobile patients. Rimantadine (Flumadine®) is a much safer choice. It can have side effects, such as convulsions, but they are rare. Reducing the dosage to below 100 mg daily is only recommended in patients with severe hepatic insufficiency. The same dose can be used for prophylaxis and therapy. However, those being treated should be separated from those who are on prophylaxis to reduce the possibility of spread of a resistant virus.

Zanamivir must be inhaled to be effective. It has been used in nursing homes, but a certain proportion of residents will not be able to inhale deeply enough to receive the full dose. They may also need help with the device. Because systematic absorption of the drug is not significant, there is little possibility of drug-drug interaction. Two inhalations once a day (a total of 10 mg of drug) are used for prophylaxis. However, zanamivir has not yet been approved for prophylaxis in the United States. The dose is given twice daily for 5 days for treatment of clinical influenza.

Because oseltamivir is taken orally, there is no need for special attention to administration. The prophylactic dose of 75 mg once a day can be given to any patient with a

14

creatinine clearance above 30 mL/min/1.73 m^2; reduction of dosage is necessary at reduced renal function. Because of the possibility of gastrointestinal intolerance, the drug should be administered with food. The dose for treatment is twice that for prophylaxis, 75 mg b.i.d., given for 5 days.

Even if there are several cases of illness at the time that control of the outbreak begins, most residents will be on prophylaxis, not therapy. Many recommendations have been made for prophylaxis duration; past recommendations have said that prophylaxis should be continued until community activity ends, which may take many weeks. Two weeks of prophylaxis is now considered adequate. Depending on the packaging of the drugs, this may be extended to 15 days. Cultures should be done during the prophylaxis period, and if more documented cases are found, the prophylaxis period should be extended another 5 to 7 days. If the M2 inhibitors are being used and it is clear that influenza is still occurring, switching to an NAI should be considered in case resistance has developed.

To avoid the development of resistance, an NAI can be used for treatment of illness and the M2 inhibitors used for prophylaxis. This is based on the fact that M2-inhibitor resistance only seems to develop during treatment. While this strategy is logical, it requires precision in identifying and isolating ill residents. It also may make writing of standing orders difficult. Whatever the details, the critical element is employment of an antiviral whenever a nursing home outbreak occurs. These outbreaks must be treated as emergencies that can cause the hospitalization and death of residents and disrupt the operation of the home.

Cruise Ship and Institutional Outbreaks

Influenza outbreaks occur regularly on cruise ships. Such outbreaks are of special concern because they can occur in the summer when vaccine is not available in the northern hemisphere. These cruises have a high proportion of older and high-risk individuals who may develop complications.[12] The outbreaks put a great burden on the ship's health-care system, which is easily overwhelmed. Control measures are similar to those for nursing homes. However, isolation and cohorting of ill individuals may be difficult because of space requirements. As in nursing homes, antivirals should be stocked on these ships because it is only through use of antivirals that an outbreak can be terminated quickly. Methods for antiviral use should be adapted from those used in nursing homes. Vaccination should be a priority for people going on cruises in the winter, when vaccine is usually available.

Other residential institutions, such as schools and camps, are common sites of influenza outbreaks. In these settings, the concern is high morbidity from extensive transmission. Residents of such institutions may be vaccinated as a method of preventing outbreaks and are specifically mentioned in Advisory Committee on Immunization Practices recommendations as a 'group to consider.' Antivirals should also be considered once an outbreak begins. Complications may be rare, but high morbidity can result in great disruption.

Health-Care Settings

Nosocomial outbreaks are often reported and are one reason vaccination recommendations target health-care workers. As noted above, certain patients, such as those with immunosuppression, are at high risk of severe infection, and they are frequently infected by staff or, sometimes, other patients. Standard infection control techniques should be put in place if cases of influenza are detected in already admitted patients. Patients admitted because of influenza create less concern because the infection has already been recognized. Antivirals have been highly successful in containing outbreaks in these situations. Health-care workers should be included in prophylaxis or therapy to contain further introduction and spread. This is usually simpler to implement than in highly transient nursing home personnel.

14

Influenza has occurred in neonatal intensive care units, sometimes out of season, creating problems in disease recognition. Again, unvaccinated staff introduce the infection. Ideally, the patients should be protected by antivirals, but there are little data on how to use oseltamivir or the M2 inhibitors in a group this young. Amantadine has been used at 5 mg/kg/day with some success. However, adverse events may be seen at this dose, and they become common at higher doses. In such settings, chronic shedding is common. It may be possible in the future to examine how oseltamivir would function in this situation, especially in terms of induction of antiviral resistance.

Pregnancy

Vaccination is recommended for women who will be pregnant during the influenza season to reduce the possibility of severe disease. Vaccination can occur during any trimester. The possibility of severe disease is greater in women with chronic underlying conditions.[13,14] Until the NAIs were developed, little could be done for such women who developed a moderate or severe case of influenza. When amantadine and rimantadine were developed, their animal toxicology was not as extensively studied as would be required today. However, the studies that were done indicate that the drugs are teratogenic and embryolethal. Therefore, they should not be given to pregnant women, especially now that the NAIs are available. Zanamivir and oseltamivir have been much more extensively studied in terms of short- and long-term toxicity, and no major abnormalities have been demonstrated, although minor skeletal changes were noted at high doses of each in laboratory animals. Both drugs are therefore classified as Category C. However, the low levels of absorption of zanamivir make it preferable for treatment of severe influenza in a woman late in her pregnancy, especially if she has an underlying condition. To avoid this problem, vaccination should be given before the season.

References

1. Lin JC, Nichol KL: Excess mortality due to pneumonia or influenza during influenza seasons among persons with acquired immunodeficiency syndrome. *Arch Intern Med* 2001;161:441-446.

2. Fine AD, Bridges CB, De Guzman AM, et al: Influenza A among patients with human immunodeficiency virus: an outbreak of infection at a residential facility in New York City. *Clin Infect Dis* 2001; 32:1784-1791.

3. Fuller JD, Craven DE, Steger KA, et al: Influenza vaccination of human immunodeficiency virus (HIV)-infected adults: impact on plasma levels of HIV type 1 RNA and determinants of antibody response. *Clin Infect Dis* 1999;28:541-547.

4. Klimov AI, Rocha E, Hayden FG, et al: Prolonged shedding of amantadine-resistant influenzae A viruses by immunodeficient patients: detection by polymerase chain reaction-restriction analysis. *J Infect Dis* 1995;172:1352-1355.

5. Englund JA, Champlin RE, Wyde PR, et al: Common emergence of amantadine- and rimantadine-resistant influenza A viruses in symptomatic immunocompromised adults. *Clin Infect Dis* 1998; 26:1418-1424.

6. Gubareva LV, Matrosovich MN, Brenner MK, et al: Evidence for zanamivir resistance in an immunocompromised child infected with influenza B virus. *J Infect Dis* 1998;178:1257-1262.

7. Zadeh MM, Buxton Bridges C, Thompson WW, et al: Influenza outbreak detection and control measures in nursing homes in the United States. *J Am Geriatr Soc* 2000;48:1310-1315.

8. Buxton JA, Skowronski DM, Ng H, et al: Influenza revaccination of elderly travelers: antibody response to single influenza vaccination and revaccination at 12 weeks. *J Infect Dis* 2001;184:188-191.

9. Ohmit SE, Arden MN, Monto AS: Effectiveness of inactivated influenza vaccine among nursing home residents during an influenza type A (H3N2) epidemic. *J Am Geriatr Soc* 1999;47:165-171.

10. Potter J, Stott DJ, Roberts MA, et al: Influenza vaccination of health care workers in long-term-care hospitals reduces the mortality of elderly patients. *J Infect Dis* 1997;175:1-6.

11. Patriarca PA, Weber JA, Parker RA, et al: Efficacy of influenza vaccine in nursing homes. Reduction in illness and complications during an influenza A (H3N2) epidemic. *JAMA* 1985;253:1136-1139.

14

12. Miller JM, Tam TW, Maloney S, et al: Cruise ships: high-risk passengers and the global spread of new influenza viruses. *Clin Infect Dis* 2000;31:433-438.

13. Freeman DW, Barno A: Deaths from Asian influenza associated with pregnancy. *Am J Obstet Gynecol* 1959;78:1172-1175.

14. Neuzil KM, Reed GW, Mitchel EF, et al: Impact of influenza on acute cardiopulmonary hospitalizations in pregnant women. *Am J Epidemiol* 1998;148:1094-1102.

Chapter 15

Pandemics: The Threat of Avian Influenza

Past pandemics have been described in Chapter 2. The overall impact of pandemics and the groups most affected by them are known and well described. However, the interval between pandemics can vary, and the impact of each pandemic depends on the infecting virus. For example, the interval between the pandemics of 1918 and 1957 was close to 40 years, followed by an interval of only 11 years to the pandemic of 1968, and the characteristics of each of these pandemics were different. The A(H3N2) pandemic of 1968 was less severe than the A(H2N2) outbreak of 1957, probably because only the viral hemagglutinin changed. The 1918 A(H1N1) outbreak was devastating. Also, the 1957 and 1968 pandemics were lethal mainly to those with underlying disease and those at the extremes of age. However, in 1918, healthy adults were also severely affected. These differences create issues in predicting when the next pandemic will occur and what its characteristics will be.

Planning on the basis of experience has been further complicated by the current avian influenza episode, which started in Hong Kong in 1997 and involved the A(H5N1) virus. This virus was probably transmitted from geese to chickens in the live-bird markets. What is certain is that

15

this virus was in the Eurasian lineage of the avian influenza virus, as described in Chapter 8. Once in the chickens, it was highly infectious and lethal, killing all the chickens on one bird farm and destroying almost 70% of the chickens on another. This outbreak occurred in March to May 1997. In May, a 3-year-old child died of a severe case of influenza. This child had an underlying disease and developed Reye's syndrome, so the death itself was not considered unusual. However, the virus isolate from the child did not type with sera for the human influenza viruses now circulating, so it was sent to a reference laboratory and identified as A(H5N1).[1] The human isolate was found to be almost identical to the avian virus, which indicated that it had been transmitted directly from birds to humans.[2] This event violated the assumption that direct interspecies transmission was impossible because of the difference in cell receptors in birds and humans. It was thought that the virus had to pass through pigs, which possess both kinds of cell receptors and can be coinfected with avian and human viruses.[3] The next step, at least in theory, would be a mixing of gene segments, known as reassortment, so that the resulting virus would carry a mixture of segments from the parent avian and human viruses. The 1957 and 1968 pandemics were caused by reassortant viruses. However, the virus that infected the child in Hong Kong was one that still had avian characteristics, not a reassortant.

An additional 17 people contracted influenza caused by this virus in November and December of 1997 and 5 died. At the same time, renewed transmission of the virus in chickens occurred, but not with the same lethality. Of the total 18 human cases, 6 died, making the case fatality an unprecedented 33%. While there were suggestions that adults fared less well than children, the small numbers made it difficult to draw conclusions. The good news was that this A(H5N1) virus did not transmit from person to person. There was evidence of a few asymptomatic infections in contacts of those who became clinically ill, but no further spread. This was further evidence that the virus was still not adapted to the human host.

Transmission of the A(H5N1) virus was still occurring among chickens in Hong Kong when infection with the usual A(H3N2) virus began in humans in early 1998, raising the possibility of reassortment in a person coinfected with the A(H5N1) and A(H3N2) viruses. Such a reassortment could result in a virus with the lethal potential of the avian virus and the potential to spread from person to person. This prospect was of such concern that the live-bird markets were 'depopulated,' which is still considered a controversial action in Hong Kong. However, no more A(H5N1) cases occurred in humans. The markets for aquatic and terrestrial birds have since been separated to reduce the possibility of viral transmission from geese to chickens. This separation seemed to work for a few years. More recently, however, the virus occasionally reappeared in poultry, although not with such extensive spread.

In 2003, separate incidents occurred in various parts of the globe with widely different consequences. In British Columbia, a massive outbreak of a highly pathogenic H7N3 virus involved poultry-raising areas of the province. To control it, millions of birds were culled, and containment was finally achieved, but at great economic cost. Little, if any, human infection could be demonstrated.[4] It was even hard to determine whether protective clothing worn by cullers had any role in protecting them because transmission to humans was so infrequent.

A massive outbreak of a highly pathogenic H7N7 virus occurred in the Netherlands and in surrounding areas. As with the British Columbia outbreak, culling was instituted and the uninfected poultry were moved to covered areas to limit exposure to migratory birds, which had probably introduced the virus. However, unlike the situation in Canada, there was evidence of moderate transmission to persons in contact with the poultry, and also sometimes to their families. There was even a death reported in a veterinarian in contact

15

with infected birds. The virus was sensitive to oseltamivir, and the drug was used extensively to prevent further spread to those in contact with the infected poultry.[5]

However, it was in Asia that the continuing extensive explosion of avian influenza began in late 2003. As before, this explosion was because of the A(H5N1) virus. A prelude occurred in the first part of the year, when two cases in humans were detected in Hong Kong after infection in the Fujian Province. Presumably, transmission in birds was occurring in that area of coastal China. At the end of the same year, the A(H5N1) virus began to cause deaths in poultry in a wide crescent from Korea and Japan in the north to Indonesia, Vietnam, and Thailand in the south. The virus spread occasionally from birds to humans, first documented in Thailand and Vietnam, and was found to be a more lethal variant than the 1997 virus and was termed the 'Z' strain. Not only did it cause more severe disease in humans, but it was resistant to the M2 inhibitors. In avian species, the spread of these viruses has continued with evidence of the developing of further variation. More recently it has arrived in Turkey and some countries in eastern Europe, as a result of infection in migrating birds.

The disease in humans caused by the 'Z' strain has not been completely documented. It is clear, however, that it produces an even more severe disease than that seen in Hong Kong in 1997. Although there is debate about whether milder cases are being missed, the reported case fatality is in excess of 50%. Recognized signs and symptoms are shown in Table 15-1.[6] They suggest that, unlike ordinary influenza, this is a disseminated infection. In animal models, such as mice and ferrets, this is clearly the case, with virus present in the spleen and brain.[7] This has implications for antiviral therapy.

Transmission of this virus to humans usually involves relatively close contact with infected birds, although there is some evidence of transmission through uncooked duck blood. Further transmission from one human to another has

Table 15-1: Characteristics of 10 Patients With Avian (H5N1) Influenza in Vietnam

Age: 5-24 years (mean 13.7 years)

Cough/Dyspnea	100%
Diarrhea	70%
Rash	0%
Conjunctivitis	0%
Fever	100%
Leukopenia	100%
Thrombocytopenia	90%
Markedly abnormal x-rays	100%
Death	80%
Oseltamivir used	50%

Tran TH, et al: *N Engl J Med* 2004;350:1179-1188

occasionally been observed. These viruses retained fully avian characteristics that would not allow them to infect humans easily. However, they could mutate or reassort, exchanging genetic information with a regular type A human strain. This would likely result in a pandemic, which, if the lethality of the virus does not moderate, would be potentially more like 1918 than 1957 or 1968.

Surveillance for Pandemic Preparation

Any plans for pandemic control require an early warning system so that appropriate actions, such as vaccine production, can take place promptly. To this end, the World Health Organization (WHO) has a surveillance network to detect influenza virus strains as they circulate around the world. Virologic surveillance is essential for the reformulation of the influenza vaccine on an annual basis. Because new interpandemic viruses have often originated in East Asia, a special effort has been mounted to increase the number of surveillance sites in that part of the world. The result of this activity is that only once in the last 10 years has a component in the vaccine not matched the circulating virus.[8]

The same issues apply to detecting pandemic viruses. There are increased numbers of sites working on influenza virus detection in areas of East Asia within and outside China. However, there are also large areas of the world, especially in much of Africa, where there is no surveillance activity at all. In the unlikely event that a new virus originates in any of these parts of the world, it may take several extra weeks for it to spread to an area with laboratories that can recognize that an outbreak is taking place.

A virus will be considered to have pandemic potential if it is a type A virus and has a hemagglutinin and possibly a neuraminidase different from that of one of the current viruses. Following the experience with the A(H5N1) virus described above and the more recent sporadic detection in humans of the avian A(H9N2) viruses in China and Hong Kong, it is clear that true human-to-human spread must be demonstrated before a pandemic alert is issued. Making the decision to issue an alert may be difficult. In 1976, disease caused by swine influenza and transmitted in military recruits triggered a pandemic alert in the United States. That decision seemed correct at the time, but perhaps planning and vaccine production should have stopped when no continued transmission was detected.[9] The WHO has produced a revised pandemic plan that proposes various stages of alert in recognition of these and similar problems.[10] The stages of alert are shown in Table 15-2. Of note is the division of the pre-pandemic stages into several levels. This is in recognition of the fact that

Table 15-2: New WHO Pandemic Phases

Interpandemic Period

Phase 1	No new type A influenza subtypes detected in humans.
Phase 2	No new type A subtypes in humans. Subtypes in animals pose substantial risk of human disease.

Pandemic Alert Period

Phase 3	Human infections with new subtype, but no human-to-human spread.
Phase 4	Small clusters of human-to-human transmission, but spread highly localized.
Phase 5	Large clusters of human-to-human transmission, but geographically limited.

Pandemic Period

Phase 6	Increased and sustained transmission in the general population.

Post-Pandemic Period

Return to the interpandemic period

Adapted from: World Health Organization: WHO global influenza preparedness plan. Geneva, Switzerland, World Health Organization, 2005.

the virus may gradually acquire the changes allowing for human to human transmission. For this reason, strategies are being considered to use antivirals to try to contain the spread of the potentially pandemic virus while it is adapting to human transmission. This would ideally extinguish the pandemic at its source.[12] Declaration of a pandemic will still depend on the judgment of a group of experts, who will have to view the situation and decide whether action should be taken.

Vaccines for Use in Pandemics

Vaccines have always been viewed as the primary method of controlling pandemic diseases. The system for producing vaccines in interpandemic years is well established, based on making a decision about viral content at a fixed date that leaves sufficient time for vaccine production. Fertile eggs, needed for vaccine production, are ordered in advance from suppliers known to be reliable. Only one inoculation of vaccine is needed in all but the youngest children.

All of these events would be different in a pandemic. First, there would be no predicting when the vaccine virus would be identified. If the virus were identified when eggs were unavailable, vaccine production would be delayed. Next would be the question of how easy the vaccine is to produce. Some influenza viruses grow poorly in eggs, and although there are methods for increasing the yield, they also take time. Yield will be critical in a pandemic because demand for the vaccine will be great. For this reason, efforts have begun to produce vaccine in acceptable cell culture. Then there is the possibility that the virus will be like A(H5N1), which cannot be replicated unchanged in hens' eggs. No production facility has the biocontainment capabilities to handle such a virus. A method has been used to change the A(H5N1) virus, so that it is no longer highly lethal. It involves treating the hemagglutinin to remove the virulent multi-basic cleavage site, and then to reassemble the entire virus using eight plasmids, one for each segment of the genome. The process is called 'reverse genetics.' The altered virus has been prepared and is now being used to prepare vaccines for evaluating their use should a pandemic occur.

On the positive side, a pandemic vaccine would only need one viral component rather than the three required in the regular vaccine. This means that three times as much vaccine could be produced. If the pandemic virus is totally new, one inoculation may not be sufficient to produce protective immunity. If two injections per person are required, twice as much vaccine would need to be produced. Even more critical would be the time needed for immunity to develop. Generally, an interval of at least 2 weeks between injections is necessary to obtain the required booster effect.

It may be possible to produce the booster effect without giving a second inoculation. For example, it was recognized during the swine influenza outbreak that the older, whole virus vaccines produced higher antibody titers in unprimed children than split vaccines. Most inactivated vaccines given today are split or subunit preparations because these preparations are less likely to produce side effects. However, most side effects of whole virus vaccines, such as fever, are mild, and in a pandemic situation, the risk-benefit ratio may warrant the use of these vaccines. The viral components that do not help produce antibody to virus hemagglutinin and neuraminidase in the whole virus vaccine seem to function as an adjuvant.[13]

A more direct approach to accelerating the booster effect would be to add an adjuvant to vaccine used during a pandemic. Alum has been evaluated for this purpose. Vaccine containing MF59, which has been developed for use in interpandemic periods as well as pandemics, has also been studied. This adjuvanted vaccine has been tested using some potential hemagglutinins of pandemic viruses and has performed better than nonadjuvanted vaccine. This vaccine, using contemporary antigens, is licensed in some European countries.[14]

When the next pandemic occurs, there will be delays in identifying the new virus and producing sufficient vaccine. Everything possible should be attempted to shorten this period. Sixteen hemagglutinins have been identified in birds and other species. It would be simple to stockpile these antigens or to prepare high-yield preparations that could more quickly produce large amounts of vaccine. However, because each hemagglutinin subtype is variable, it is possible that the stockpiled antigen would not match the hemagglutinin of the circulating subtype. If the circulating virus is different from the virus in the vaccine, the vaccine will not be very effective, even if it contains the appropriate hemagglutinin subtype. Reagents for identifying new pandemic viruses are clearly needed. Delays are more likely if the antiserum required to identify the virus is unavailable. These reagents are therefore a high priority in any pandemic plan.

Antivirals for Pandemics

M2 Inhibitors

The ability to produce vaccine in sufficient quantities to control the first wave of a pandemic is of great concern. Unlike vaccine, which must contain an antigen similar or identical to that of the pandemic virus, both classes of antivirals, the M2 inhibitors and the neuraminidase inhibitors (NAIs), are effective against all type A viruses, as long as they are susceptible to drugs, which possess the M2 protein and one of the nine recognized neuraminidases. Why, then, have the antivirals generally not a prominent part of a pandemic plan? The answer is one of logistics, not lack of effectiveness. Attention has now been given to overcoming these logistic problems. The main question is which of the antivirals should be used and for what purpose: prophylaxis or therapy. Most of the current A(H5N1) avian viruses are resistant to M2 inhibitors, but these drugs are discussed here in the event this pattern changes.

Amantadine (Symmetrel®) and rimantadine (Flumadine®) are as effective in prophylaxis as the NAIs, and, based solely on their lower costs, they would appear to be the most logical choice for this purpose. However, antivirals must be given on a daily basis, raising the issue of supply. Also, amantadine produces side effects related to the central nervous system in 5% to 10% of recipients. If it were used as extensively as would be required in a pandemic, many people would experience these side effects and might put themselves or others in danger on the job and on the road. Rimantadine, which does not produce such side effects, would therefore be the M2 inhibitor of choice.[15]

Rimantadine has been shown to produce antiviral resistance. This has not been a problem in purely prophylactic situations. However, in a pandemic situation, when there would be great demand for antivirals, rimantidine would inevitably be used for treatment. This would predictably result in selection and shedding of transmissible M2-inhibitor-resistant variants.[16] Thus, it seems appropriate to plan to use the M2 inhibitors for prophylaxis as part of the overall strategy to control a pandemic of susceptible virus, using the NAIs for treatment. The dose could be 100 mg daily because there is reasonable evidence that these drugs work in prophylaxis at such a dosage. This is half of the approved dosage, except in the nursing home elderly, and it would need to be tested and approved as part of development of a pandemic plan. Halving the dose would double the numbers of individuals who could be put on prophylaxis.

Neuraminidase Inhibitors

Zanamivir (Relenza®) and oseltamivir (Tamiflu®) could be used for prophylaxis and therapy, but they will probably be reserved for treatment. Their ability to prevent complications would make them particularly important in treating cases of pandemic influenza.[17] They can also shorten the duration of illness, which is important in older persons and persons with more severe disease[18] and, in a pandemic, will be critical in getting persons who provide vital community services back to work as soon as possible. However, prevention of lower respiratory complications would be

213

enough to justify the use of NAIs in the pandemic situation because these complications can result in hospitalization and death, and use of the NAIs may lower the frequency of those outcomes.

Because A(H5N1) disease in humans appears to be a disseminated infection, oseltamivir has been favored for stockpiling. Who should be recommended to receive antivirals will therefore be an issue if, as expected, the NAIs are in short supply. Most severe complications of pandemic illness occur in older individuals; however, very young children, patients with underlying chronic conditions, and even healthy adults have higher proportional mortality rates during pandemics than in interpandemic outbreaks. Also, the reduction of complications seems to be greater in younger adults than in the elderly. This does not mean that older individuals with illness should not be treated. The contrary is true. What it does suggest is that previously healthy younger adults may also warrant treatment.

Current recommendations are 5 days of treatment. However, since all are naïve to a pandemic virus, and because, for example, with A(H5N1) infection, replication in humans and experimental animals occurs for more than 5 days, longer treatment may be necessary.[7] Resistance has not been a problem with the NAIs, and this is clearly different from the situation with the M2 inhibitors. However, with more extensive use this might change. Fortunately, the amino acid substitution sometimes seen with N1 viruses produces a virus resistant to oseltamivir but not zanamivir.

Vaccines and Antivirals: Complementary Use in Pandemic Planning

A pandemic plan has been developed for the US and billions of dollars recommended to fund vaccine development and stockpiling of antivirals. Among the strategies to improve vaccine availability will be to develop them in cell culture. There are also plans to investigate methods, such as use of adjuvants to reduce the amount of antigen required to produce an immune response, thus increasing the amount that can be produced with a limited supply of viral product.

Vaccines would be the ideal choice for control of pandemics. However, vaccine production will likely be delayed and there will not be enough vaccine available for all who wish to be vaccinated. A policy will need to be put in place to prioritize use of vaccine. Mathematical simulations based on various amounts of vaccine being available have been used to examine this issue. One recommended strategy relies on vaccination of school-aged children as a method of reducing overall transmission. However, it is more likely that the priorities recommended for pandemic use will be similar to those used when normal vaccine production is delayed. This order of vaccination stresses those who are at the highest risk and health-care workers. Some countries, such as Switzerland, put vaccination of health-care workers first in their pandemic plan, on the principle that they need to remain healthy to care for others. This could change if, as in 1918, younger individuals are the ones most affected.

Similarly, the use of antivirals, especially for prophylaxis, will depend on whether and how much vaccine is available. Antivirals for prophylaxis must be taken every day, but they can be used in the face of the pandemic because, unlike vaccines, they do not require time for the recipient to build immunity. Health-care workers and others essential to community activities might be considered to receive antiviral prophylaxis. Prophylactic antivirals might also be considered for those at highest risk of complications if no vaccine is available. However, in the current situation, with only oseltamivir and zanamivir being stockpiled, most will be used for treatment. With regard to treatment, administration of antivirals must be initiated early in the illness. All those in certain high-risk groups could be treated.

15

Many difficult issues of prioritization could be reduced if antiviral stockpiles are large enough. The size of stockpiles is now limited by production capacity and funds appropriated for purchase. The stability of the drugs themselves is not an issue. Shelf life has been extended as more time has elapsed for evaluation. Given the potential impact of a pandemic, especially one caused by A(H5N1), the costs of a stockpile and for vaccine research would seem worthwhile. Much of the vaccine research could help in developing new approaches to prevention, that is, to an improved vaccine.

References

1. Subbarao K, Kilmov A, Katz J, et al: Characterization of an avian influenza A (H5N1) virus isolated from a child with a fatal respiratory illness. *Science* 1998;279:393-396.

2. Claas EC, Osterhaus AD, van Beek R, et al: Human influenza A H5N1 virus related to a highly pathogenic avian influenza virus. *Lancet* 1998;351:472-477.

3. Scholtissek C: Pigs as 'mixing vessels' for the creation of new pandemic influenza A viruses. *Med Princ Pract* 1990;2:65-71.

4. Tweed SA, Skowronski DM, David ST, et al: Human illness from avian influenza H7N3, British Columbia. *Emerg Infect Dis* 2004;10:2196-2199.

5. Koopmans M, Wilbrink B, Conyn M, et al: Transmission of H7N7 avian influenza A virus to human beings during a large outbreak in commercial poultry farms in the Netherlands. *Lancet* 2004;363:587-593.

6. Hien TT, Nguyen TL, Nguyen TD, et al: Avian influenza A(H5N1) in 10 patients in Vietnam. *N Engl J Med* 2004;350:1179-1188.

7. Yen HL, Monto AS, Webster RG, et al: Virulence may determine the necessary duration and dosage of oseltamivir treatment for highly pathogenic A/Vietnam/1203/04 (H5N1) influenza virus in mice. *J Infect Dis* 2005;192:665-672.

8. Shortridge KF, Stuart-Harris CH: An influenza epicentre? *Lancet* 1982;2:812-813.

9. Weinstein L: Influenza—1918, a revisit? [editorial]. *N Engl J Med* 1976;294:1058-1060.

10. World Health Organization (WHO): Influenza pandemic preparedness plan: the role of WHO and guidelines for national and regional planning. Geneva: WHO, 1999. WHO/CDS/CSR/EDC/99.1.

11. World Health Organization: WHO global influenza preparedness plan. Geneva, Switzerland: World Health Organization; 2005. Available at: http://www.who.int/csr/resources/publications/influenza/WHO_CDS_CSR_GIP_2005_5/en/index.html. Accessed May 9, 2005.

12. Monto AS: The threat of an avian influenza pandemic. *N Engl J Med* 2005;352:323-325.

13. Wright PF, Thompson J, Vaughn WK, et al: Trials of influenza A/New Jersey/76 virus vaccine in normal children: an overview of age-related antigenicity and reactogenicity. *J Infect Dis* 1977; 136(suppl): S731-S741.

14. Nicholson KG, Colegate AE, Podda A, et al: Safety and antigenicity of non-adjuvanted and MF59-adjuvanted influenza A/Duck/Singapore/97 (H5N3) vaccine: a randomised trial of two potential vaccines against H5N1 influenza. *Lancet* 2001;357:1937-1943.

15. Keyser LA, Karl M, Nafziger AN, et al: Comparison of central nervous system adverse effects of amantadine and rimantadine used as sequential prophylaxis of influenza A in elderly nursing home patients. *Arch Intern Med* 2000;160:1485-1488.

16. Mast EE, Harmon MW, Gravenstein S, et al: Emergence and possible transmission of amantadine-resistant viruses during nursing home outbreaks of influenza A (H3N2). *Am J Epidemiol* 1991;134:988-997.

17. Kaiser L, Keene ON, Hammond JM, et al: Impact of zanamivir on antibiotic use for respiratory events following acute influenza in adolescents and adults. *Arch Intern Med* 2000;160:3234-3240.

18. Monto AS, Moult AB, Sharp SJ: Effect of zanamivir on duration and resolution of influenza symptoms. *Clin Ther* 2000;22:1294-1305.

15

Chapter **16**

Current Practice

T
he current approach for the control of influenza should involve a combined use of vaccine and antivirals. The inactivated vaccine remains the principal method for preventing influenza. However, the United States has had a paradoxical situation during the last few years with the current vaccine. Just as a new large group, individuals from 50 to 64 years of age, was added to the risk category recommended for vaccination, the first year of vaccine shortage or delay occurred. The new recommendation did not create the problem but complicated it. It is, in reality, as much a problem of supply as one of demand. The number of suppliers of vaccine in the United States had decreased, while the demand was increasing. There are many explanations for this phenomenon. One of the likely reasons is that, unlike most pharmaceuticals, influenza vaccine was priced lower in North America than in many other parts of the world. Therefore, many global manufacturers do not import vaccine into the United States because of the increased global demand for vaccine, particularly in newly industrialized countries. This trend has ended, with additional manufacturers bringing vaccine to the US.

Priorities for Inactivated Vaccine Use

As a result of delays in the vaccine supply each autumn, the Advisory Committee on Immunization Practices has devised a list of priorities within those who are recommended to receive vaccine. This has complicated a situation that used to be simple. It used to be said that anyone who wants protection against influenza in a particular year should be given vaccine because there are few contraindications. With shortages, the concern is that giving the vaccine to healthy adults, for example, might deny vaccine to an elderly person with underlying conditions or to a nursing home resident. Complicating this situation still further is the fact that different groups of medical caregivers provide vaccine to different patients, so they cannot easily prioritize what supplies they have. In the past, the manufacturers have not been able to send vaccine in the preferential direction because of 'middlemen' being involved. This deficiency has been at least partially corrected. Still, the ultimate solution would be to increase the supply of vaccine in the United States and to increase early availability. Ways must be found for those older than 64 years, those with chronic conditions, nursing home residents, and health-care personnel to receive vaccine before even an early influenza season. The addition of Fluarix® to the available vaccines is evidence that shortages may soon be a thing of the past.

Influenza vaccine must be administered yearly in order to be effective. This is the case not only because the viruses may be changed to match those circulating, but also because antibody levels fall fairly rapidly after inoculation. This fact has led to two questionable practices. The first practice is a delay in the administration of the vaccine to a time just before the influenza season, which assumes that there is an adequate supply of vaccine. While this is possible, given sufficient timely vaccine supplies for individuals in institutions, it may result in a lack of vaccination for persons who live independently and need vaccine. The basic rule is to vaccinate such individuals whenever they have contact with the health-care system. The second questionable practice is the revaccination of those individuals who have been vaccinated early; this would occur when the outbreak is delayed. This was al-

16

ways discouraged, and a recent study indicates that it is ineffective in producing higher antibody levels.

Live-Attenuated Vaccines

The American live-attenuated influenza vaccine (LAIV) is now available in the United States. This will make it possible to vaccinate segments of the population not traditionally given the inactivated vaccine. Children under 5 years of age cannot be given this vaccine, but that may change after current studies are completed. Immunizing healthy children reduces the transmission of influenza in the community. An estimated 70% of school-age children need to be vaccinated for this phenomenon to be demonstrated; however, there may be lesser effects produced where fewer children are vaccinated. In the studies in the former Soviet Union with the Russian vaccine, an effect was seen in protecting unvaccinated teachers and other students at lower vaccination frequency. Studies examining this issue need to be continued, and, now that an LAIV has been licensed, proper observations need to be made. A question in vaccinating school-aged children will be the sustainability of such a program. Many of our problems with inactivated influenza vaccine would disappear if we did not have to vaccinate annually. Annual vaccination is also required with the live-attenuated vaccines.

Use of Antivirals in Prophylaxis

Vaccines are our first line of protection against influenza. They are relatively inexpensive, and protection lasts for much of the influenza season. Vaccine efficacy in healthy adults is approximately 70% to 90%. In older individuals with underlying conditions, efficacy is lower, especially in the nursing home elderly. It is also lower in those rare situations in which the virus in the vaccine is not similar to the circulating strain. That situation last occurred in 1997-1998, when A/Sydney(H3N2) began circulating after the vaccine that contained A/Wuhan(H3N2) had been distributed. Any situation in which vaccine efficacy is low would be one in which antiviral prophylaxis should be considered, at least for certain categories of individuals. Because it requires daily administration of a drug, seasonal prophylaxis with antivirals is not usually a strong consideration, except when a new variant not represented in the vaccine spreads. In this case, it could be considered for individuals with risk conditions and those who need protection because of their occupations, such as health-care workers. It is important to recognize early that with a new variant, little protection from the current vaccine in reducing morbidity and mortality is taking place. The situation has some of the characteristics of a pandemic with short vaccine supplies.

In years when there is a good match between the circulating strain and the strain in the vaccine, seasonal prophylaxis could be considered among frail nursing home elderly, especially when A(H3N2) viruses are circulating. Such administration adds significantly to the overall probability that an individual in a nursing home will be protected, but, because of cost issues, it will rarely be used. It should, however, be strongly considered if the virus circulating has changed significantly from the one in the vaccine. There were many nursing home outbreaks in the year in which A/Sydney circulated. However, for most years, the major strategy in nursing homes will be outbreak control (see Chapter 15).

The main indication for seasonal antiviral prophylaxis annually would be for the small number of individuals who, because of egg allergies, cannot receive the vaccine. These individuals often have asthma or underlying conditions that put them in the high-risk classification. Travelers and individuals on cruises, especially at times when vaccine is not available, might also benefit from seasonal use of the drugs, but only when they are at risk.

A special case is an unvaccinated patient with a risk condition, who is encountered by a medical caregiver when influenza is transmitting. That person should be vaccinated and put on an antiviral for at least 2 weeks while antibody to the vaccination is developing. Antivirals will not inhibit the response to the inactivated vaccine.

Postexposure Prophylaxis

Most prophylactic use of antivirals will be targeted (ie, for a period of weeks). When one individual in the household or the workplace becomes ill with influenza, there is a heightened risk that another in the household or workplace will become affected. The studies on postexposure prophylaxis are described in Chapters 12 and 13. In general, the method would be to put the first, or index, case on drug and the potential contacts on prophylaxis, using an appropriate antiviral. Prophylaxis would be used for 10 to 15 days. The longer period would protect against new exposures from the community. Generally, when these household outbreaks are recognized, the outbreak is raging in the community, and new introductions are likely to happen until the outbreak has begun to wane.

Choice of Antiviral for Prophylaxis

M2 inhibitors and neuraminidase inhibitors (NAIs) are equally effective in seasonal prophylaxis in open populations. However, unless it is clear that the influenza strain circulating is a type A virus, the NAIs would have to be used. Resistance to the M2 inhibitors has limited their use sharply. At present, oseltamivir (Tamiflu™) is the only NAI approved for prophylaxis. For seasonal prophylaxis, the preferred M2 inhibitor would clearly be rimantadine (Flumadine®) because of its better safety profile. In closed or semiclosed populations, such as households in which the index case is being treated, the NAIs would be the clear choice. Prophylaxis has failed in this situation because of the selection of resistant variants by both amantadine (Symmetrel®) and rimantadine.

Treatment With Antivirals

The questions that arise when considering treatment are which cases should be treated and how they should be identified. The first question can be answered by turning the issue around to the use of antibiotics for streptococcal pharyngitis. In this case, all would treat with antibiotics, not only to shorten the duration of the illness, but also to prevent complications. For the same reason, anyone with an influenza illness serious enough to present to a physician should be considered for antiviral treatment. Duration of illness will be shortened, with improvement beginning within one day of the start of therapy. The more severe the illness is, the more dramatic the effect of therapy. Complications requiring antibiotics will also be prevented, including otitis media in children and bronchitis and pneumonia in adults. All of these findings have been demonstrated with both of the NAIs, with the exception of the otitis media reduction, which has been found only with oseltamivir. The decision to treat should be made as quickly as possible because, after onset, earlier treatment leads to a greater benefit.

The second question is how to recognize that the case is an influenza infection. There are now several rapid antigen detection tests available; however, a problem in use on an individual basis is that they are often of relatively low sensitivity (one recent study demonstrated a sensitivity of approximately 40%) and have been known to be nonspecific. The sensitivity may vary from test to test; this variability may also be a reflection of the type of specimens and the way that they are collected.

The large clinical trials of zanamivir (Relenza®) and oseltamivir all used clinical criteria to determine who had influenza, with a critical proviso; there had to be laboratory-confirmed transmission of influenza occurring in the area. As a result, in a number of studies, 65% to 70% of those recruited were found to have influenza. Further studies have shown that it is important to know

16

when influenza viruses are present in the community. Then, if a patient with suspect influenza on the basis of clinical characteristics has cough and fever, between 79% and 87% of individuals will have influenza. A higher temperature indicates a greater likelihood that the case will be influenza (Figure 1). This exceeds the sensitivity of most of the rapid tests, which can be used to identify influenza within minutes. In addition, the rapid tests will add costs to the treatment of an ill individual. Situations in which rapid antigen detection tests would aid in the recognition of whether the case is influenza would be in young individuals, where disease characteristics are not as clear, and in the first patients of a nursing home outbreak, to confirm that an agent such as respiratory syncytial virus, which sometimes causes similar outbreaks, is not responsible. Hospitalized individuals present a special case, where techniques such as a polymerase chain reaction assay might be useful in making an absolute diagnosis. Special consideration might be given to identification of a type A virus versus a type B virus, if use of an M2 inhibitor is planned.

Choice of Drugs for Therapy

Prevention of complications with amantadine and rimantadine has not been demonstrated; therefore, the NAIs would clearly be the first choice in therapy. This would especially be the case if there are mixed type A and type B outbreaks or if type B is involved. Resistance to the M2 inhibitors of type A viruses has made their use problematic. In treating an individual case, the issue of M2-inhibitor-induced resistance would not be relevant, except in a closed population, but the lack of evidence on complications would seem persuasive. Zanamivir and oseltamivir appear equivalent in older children and adults. However, for zanamivir, care would need to be given to ensure that the patient can use the inhalation device. It is relatively simple but may require some instruction.

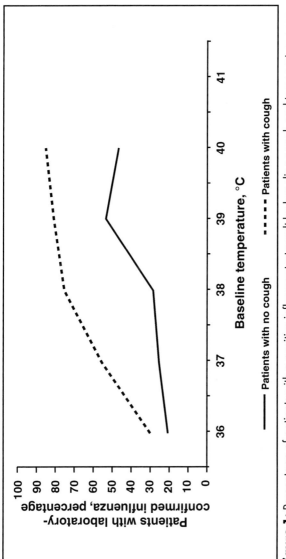

Figure 1: Percentage of patients with a positive influenza test result by baseline cough and temperature score. Monto et al, *Arch Intern Med* 2000;160:3243-3247.

Conclusions

Now that we are in the 21st century, we are beginning to see a profound change taking place in the recognition and control of influenza. Some, but not all, of this interest results from fear that avian influenza might spread to humans. Seasonal influenza is now recognized for what it is, a threat to public health in all years, but especially if pandemics occur. Until recently, our major interventions for prevention and treatment were an inactivated vaccine introduced in the 1940s and antivirals developed in the 1960s. Now we have new antivirals and new vaccines, as well as others in development. Other new interventions are in the pipeline. With these weapons, we are now in a position to make a real difference in the management of a potentially deadly disease. All it takes is planning, recognition, and prompt action.

Index

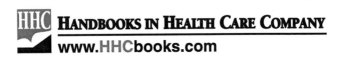
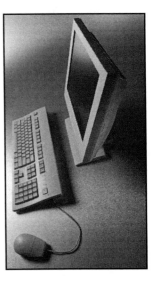